W9-BCS-184

The Galveston Diet

The Galveston Diet

The Doctor-Developed, Patient-Proven Plan to Burn Fat and Tame Your Hormonal Symptoms

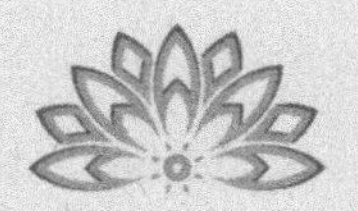

Mary Claire Haver, MD

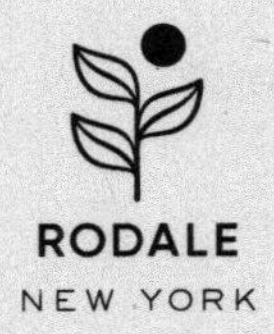

RODALE
NEW YORK

No book can replace the diagnostic expertise and medical advice of a trusted physician. Please be certain to consult with your doctor before making any decisions that affect your health, particularly if you suffer from any medical conditions or have any symptoms that may require treatment.

Published in the United States by Rodale Books, an imprint of Random House, a division of Penguin Random House LLC, New York.

RodaleBooks.com

RandomHouseBooks.com

Library of Congress Cataloging-in-Publication Data has been applied for.

ISBN 978-0-593-57889-6

Ebook ISBN 978-0-593-57890-2

Printed in the United States of America

Book design by Andrea Lau
Jacket design by Anna Bauer Carr
Jacket photograph by lingqi xie/Getty Images

10 9

First Edition

To every patient, friend, coworker, student, and follower who said,
"Help me, I don't understand what is happening to me."

CONTENTS

The Galveston Diet

INTRODUCTION

From our first day of life until the last, our bodies are always changing. This is a part of aging—a natural process no one can escape. But the changes that happen to women in midlife are unique and are often unsettling. Suddenly we're having odd symptoms like hot flashes and an accumulation of strange, new weight gain around our midsections. Our skin can be very dry or wrinkling more. We may have joint pain, hair loss, headaches, bloating, and worsening anxiety or depression. Sleep becomes elusive. Sexual intercourse can hurt. Little things set us off.

A lot of this may be happening to you right now. Trust me, you are not alone. Let me introduce you to someone who knows exactly what you're going through: me.

I was a busy physician, a mom, and a wife in my late forties. My main health challenge at the time was polycystic ovary syndrome (PCOS), a condition caused by insulin resistance, in which insulin can't do its job of ushering glucose into cells for energy. PCOS leads to erratic periods, acne, infertility, ovarian cysts, and unwanted hair growth.

About 1 in 10 women of childbearing age has PCOS. The majority (about 70 percent) are overweight or even obese, but I was among the 30 percent of normal weight. Fortunately, PCOS is treatable, and in my case, taking hormones greatly helped.

Then came a death in my family; I lost my brother, Bob, to liver failure. I was despondent. He was my daughters' favorite uncle, a creative fun spirit with whom I had a special bond. We were dance partners when I was younger, winning dance competitions all over Louisiana. When he died, I was heartbroken, and losing him brought crushing pain.

Grief does strange things to each of us. For me, I coped by bingeing. Night after night after long clinic shifts, I stood in front of my pantry, gobbling handfuls of Goldfish crackers. I'd wash them down with glasses of wine. Pretty quickly I gained nearly 20 pounds. I looked like a different person, and I felt miserable.

With my medical background, I knew that at my age it might be time to come off the hormones for a while. So, I talked to my own doctor, and we agreed that I should.

But taking the hormones had masked the perimenopausal symptoms that occur during midlife, so within two weeks of being off them, everything abruptly changed—and not for the better. I had hot flashes and I felt like I was burning from the inside out. Along came sleepless nights and, most troubling of all, the fuzzy and forgetful feeling called brain fog. My long, thick hair started falling out by the brushful. My skin felt parched from head to toe, and I had to completely change my skincare routine to keep my skin moisturized. My body ached so much that I kidded with a friend that I'd give up my firstborn to get relief. My sleep became a recurring nightmare of multiple awakenings through the night—at first drenched in sweat, and then freezing once the hot flash passed.

I knew I was going through a period of hormonal change—perimenopause—but the symptoms it produced were so profoundly intense that I was really alarmed. All this *on top* of the weight gain? I was a mess.

PART I

THE PROMISE

Then I heard my brother Bob's voice in my head. "Girl, you don't have to wallow in this anymore. You got yourself into this; you can get yourself out."

I went to work on my weight first. I did exactly what I and other doctors had always counseled patients to do: eat less, exercise more.

My efforts paid off, sort of. I'd lose a pound or two, but that was it. Then the weight would come right back on. I was starving myself and working out obsessively, but hardly dropping any weight. It was very frustrating. I just wanted to fix me, but nothing I did or tried was sticking.

I realized that I was struggling with the same weight issues many of my patients had told me about. They would sit in the examining room, often clutching paper gowns, and ask for advice about losing weight, frustrated with the fact that they had changed their diet and exercise habits and yet the scale kept moving in the wrong direction. I'd spend the next several minutes speaking with them about the combined power of diet and exercise. But for the majority of these women at this age, what I had been taught, and what had worked for me in the past, stopped working. They had fought for years to shed stubborn weight, without much permanent success. I'm sorry that it took having this same thing happen to me to change my tune, but that's the truth. When my own good advice didn't help me, it really hit me that I was doing something wrong.

I then threw myself into researching weight management and human metabolism—specifically as they relate to women. Medical school and my OB-GYN residency had taught us "calories in/calories out" as the only way, but clearly there had to be another. I didn't have all the answers, but I wanted them—so I could feel better myself and then I could guide and teach women how to reach the weight, the energy level, and the good health they want and deserve. I yearned to understand why we have such a tough time losing weight and keeping it off, especially as we approach and enter midlife.

My deep passion for finding answers, combined with motivation and determination, took me to some unexpected and exciting places. What kept popping up in the research were three themes: intermittent fasting, anti-inflammatory nutrition to help manage our hormonal changes, and important new science on the exact ratios of protein, carbohydrates, and fat we need to consume to burn fat.

Could these be the keys?

I decided to create my own plan using these three principles. That's when my individual health journey began. I tried out the newly minted diet on myself first. I focused on timing first and then gradually started intermittent fasting. After I mastered that, I focused on content: I began to eat more protein and fiber. I used olive oil, avocado, nuts, and seeds as my principal sources of fat. I steered clear of refined, processed carbohydrates (no more Goldfish crackers!). I restricted foods and ingredients like artificial colors and flavors that promote inflammation and disrupt the gut. What I *never* did was *count calories.* Next, I further refined the macronutrient percentages to supply more fat, moderate amounts of protein, and fewer carbohydrates.

Within several months, I lost those 20 pounds—especially around my abdomen. I was ecstatic but quickly realized the weight loss was just a pleasant side effect. More important, I felt healthier, stronger, and more energetic. My hot flashes dramatically diminished, and I was sleeping better.

I was on to something, so I asked my friends to try it. As I had been, they also were amazed about the pounds and inches they were losing. Best of all, they agreed this was easy. We didn't feel hungry all the time. No cravings. No terrible feelings of deprivation or restriction.

Next, I made copies of this three-tiered plan and handed them out to my patients. There were the same results: weight loss, fewer menopause symptoms, and more energy. Plus, they were keeping the lost pounds off, something they'd never been able to do on any of their many previous diets.

After seeing these success stories, I felt it was time to share my plan with a wider audience. I launched the initial program on Facebook for free and asked volunteers to try it. Word then spread that people were losing significant amounts of weight, including belly fat. I then wanted everyone to have access to its secrets and experience its success.

I further formalized the plan and took it to an even broader audience through an online program. Not sure of what would happen, I noticed that women began enrolling in the plan, week after week, and we were off and running. I have to admit, I was astonished to see how popular the program had become in such a short time. It was the medical diet everyone was talking about.

Enrollment in the program further skyrocketed, and to date, the plan has now helped tens of thousands of women shed unwanted pounds, shrink their waistlines, and improve their health.

I named my diet after Galveston, a coastal resort town in Texas. Although I wasn't born there, my husband and I have raised our daughters in Galveston. I call it home, and it is where I've spent much of my medical career. Now it is the birthplace of *The Galveston Diet*!

After the program took off, I wanted to further sharpen my nutrition knowledge. I enrolled in the prestigious Culinary Medicine Program at Tulane University, in Louisiana. It educates and trains doctors and other medical professions to understand and apply medical nutrition principles in a practical manner. That way, we can help our patients with nutritional modifications that improve their health.

Sixty hours of coursework and many hands-on labs later, I was certified in 2019 as a Culinary Medicine Specialist. The experience solidified and affirmed that I was on the right path with what I had developed for *The Galveston Diet*, particularly the importance of anti-inflammatory nutrition. The course also emphasized something that really stuck with me: *Nutrition is the most under-utilized medication, yet it is the most effective.*

So here I am today, humbled and gratified that so many women are *finally* achieving what they've always wanted: a beautifully fit body on the outside and an incredibly healthy one on the inside.

The Galveston Diet and You

This book expands my online program with new information and strategies. These new features include help for detoxing from sugar, new insights into menopause issues, the importance of certain under-appreciated nutrients, new science behind how macronutrients support midlife health, completely new recipes, brand-new meal plans, a maintenance plan, and other information you can't get online.

Even if you've worked through the online program, this book will be a helpful guide and resource for you as you continue your Galveston Diet journey. And if you're new to my program, welcome! You now have an opportunity to gain a 360-degree experience to achieve long-term weight loss and make a happy, healthy transition through perimenopause and menopause to postmenopause.

And, for both new and online students, this book will help you get to know your body and teach you how to treat it like a loving friend. You'll achieve peace of mind, knowing how to form new habits that give you joy and better health, and that work with your body to make you look strong, lean, and beautiful.

My plan is not the typical diet—the 21 or 30 days and you're done approach that you see so often now. Not at all! Although many women come to the program to lose weight safely and steadily, my main goal is that you use it every single day *permanently*—a total lifestyle change.

With that goal in mind and staying true to the principles that worked so well for me initially, I have designed three components of *The Galveston Diet*. They are essentially health-promoting actions that make the program work for you because they lead to good habit formation. All habits are built from actions, learning, and repetition, so that the behavior becomes automatic. In other words, you do it without much thinking. To develop good habits, you'll work on these three actions at the same time:

1. Intermittent fasting. This practice has enormous benefits for women in terms of hormone balance, metabolism, and lowering inflammation.

Of all the components of the program, this is the one that moves the needle for most women. They've told me they felt best after learning how to fast intermittently.

On the Galveston Diet, you'll do something called the 16:8 form of intermittent fasting: 16 hours of fasting with an eating window of 8 hours. I prefer this method because the fasting window is overnight. That means you sleep for many of those 16 hours (ideally half of them)! So, it becomes an easy habit to form.

2. Anti-inflammatory nutrition. The underlying issue in many diseases, chronic inflammation triggers weight gain. But weight gain also triggers inflammation, so they feed off each other in a crazy cycle. Inflammation tends to get worse in women as we age and experience menopausal hormone fluctuations. A lot of the foods we eat don't help, either, because they create inflammation throughout the body. Yet it doesn't have to be this way. There are many foods that actually fight inflammation. *The Galveston Diet* focuses on limiting the pro-inflammatory foods and increasing the anti-inflammatory foods.

3. Fuel refocus. For consistent, lasting weight loss, your body must shift its energy usage to rely more on fat as its fuel, rather than on glucose (which is generally supplied by carb-heavy diets). If you don't burn all the glucose you have in your bloodstream, the excess is stored as body fat. This metabolic fact led me to create a nutritional protocol made up of 70 percent healthy fats, 20 percent lean protein, and 10 percent quality carbohydrates. This ratio accomplishes three major metabolic feats: It encourages the body to burn fat. It trains the body to break the addiction to sugar and processed carbs. And it refocuses your eating on healthy sources of fats, protein, and carbohydrates.

Later, as you're ready to start maintenance, I'll introduce you to the Galveston Diet for Life program, in which you gradually decrease the fat percentage and increase the carbohydrate percentage, ultimately stabilizing at 40 percent fat, 20 percent protein, and 40 percent carbohydrates for lifetime success.

By the time you're well into all three actions, your body is beginning to burn fat more easily, and it will stop depositing fat in undesirable places like your abdomen. Accordingly, you could lose a tremendous amount of weight on the program. Kelli is a good example. She started the Galveston Diet and stuck with it, month after month. She ended up losing 100 pounds! She also trimmed $14^1/_2$ inches off her waist and $9^1/_2$ inches off her hips. But along with the weight loss, Kelli also noticed dramatic improvements in her sleep patterns, energy level, and digestive function, as well as decreased menopausal symptoms like hot flashes and a greater feeling of overall wellness.

Here's the big secret behind why the Galveston Diet is so effective: All three components work together synergistically to give you the best results. You have to intermittent-fast to lower inflammation and start to burn fat. You can't just fast, and still eat the standard American diet of inflammatory foods, then expect to burn fat and keep it off. You have to nourish your body with a great variety of anti-inflammatory foods. And you have to refocus your macronutrient choices to include more fat, moderate protein, and healthy carbohydrates.

Maybe you're wondering how long this diet takes to return you to great health? Well, the answer is pretty simple: There is no set amount of time; everyone loses weight and regains health at a different pace. But more important than that, remember and understand that the Galveston Diet is not a *diet* in the conventional sense of the word. It is a lifestyle.

Please don't be discouraged that this is a forever plan. Once you learn to live and eat this way, it becomes second nature to do so, and those old, health-harming habits—of reaching for fast food or sugar-laden carbs all the time—will become things of the past.

Yes, the Galveston Diet starts with a tightly orchestrated four-week plan to help you change the way you eat, but that is only the beginning. To help you stay with it *forever,* you'll transition to the Galveston Diet for Life program, which I cover in the final chapter. Most books present nutrition plans that are short term, with no guidance on what to do after you've followed the plan for several weeks. They leave you hanging, tempted to return to your old, unhealthy ways of eating (along with a frustrating return of pounds!). But with this maintenance program, that won't happen. It is a plan that shows you how to put additional anti-inflammatory foods back into your lifestyle, change your macro percentages to include less fat and more carbohydrates, and use intermittent fasting as the powerful weight-maintaining tool that it is.

Keep in mind that the word *diet* comes from the Greek word *dieta,* meaning "to live normally." However, nowadays the word mostly refers to cutting calories, even entire food groups, to help weight loss rather than a way to enjoy food and health. *The Galveston Diet* will help you lose weight and keep it off for sure, and this is critically important to health because weight gain contributes to many chronic and serious conditions in women. But the Galveston Diet, along with its maintenance plan, is primarily an eating pattern in the original sense of the world—a way of life—that promotes long-lasting health.

If you follow the Galveston Diet and change the way you live, you'll ultimately find, like I did, that weight loss is only one great benefit. (By the way, you can do this plan even if you are happy with your weight. I'm at a healthy weight now, and I live this way all the time.) There are so many more benefits besides weight loss: fewer menopause symptoms, blood sugar control, normalized blood lipid ranges, quality sleep, better gut health, greater energy, smoother skin, and more. You'll just feel better overall. Remember, *The Galveston Diet* is not a temporary stop on your journey. It is the journey! There may be ups and downs. You may take a few steps back before you charge ahead, but that's okay. This is ultimately a forward journey, and you're on this path to take better care of you. Just solidly commit yourself to moving down this path, and you will see your life and health change. I'm so happy to be on this journey with you.

Mary Claire Haver, MD

CHAPTER 1

Your Changing Body, Your Changing Needs

To say that my own transition from perimenopause to menopause was grueling would be an understatement. It turned out to be hell, pure and simple—with hot flashes, night sweats, thinning hair, dry skin, and weight gain. I was so ready to be done with it all.

But now that I look back, I see things that were not clear to me at the time. I wish I had known, for example, that symptoms can begin in your thirties, that if I had started hormone replacement therapy earlier, I could have been a whole lot more comfortable, and that mental states like moodiness, depression, or anxiety do not mean we're crazy!

Yes, your body is changing, but this is a normal part of life that all of us women go through—mainly brought on by hormonal fluctuations. This time of physical flux is categorized as three stages: perimenopause, menopause, and postmenopause. We experience these in unique ways. Let's take a look at what happens in each stage.

Perimenopause

In your mid- to late thirties or early forties, it may seem like your body is morphing right before your eyes. You may notice—and be irritated by—the discovery that your clothes don't fit as well as they used to, even if you haven't gained any weight. Your skin becomes drier. A few wrinkles are visible. You look and feel more tired than when you were younger. It's like seeing a stranger in the mirror.

If these changes are happening to you, you're most likely entering the first stage of hormonal fluctuation—perimenopause. This is a natural period of transition that begins several years before menopause. It can last from a few months to up to 10 years prior to menopause, and it is your body's natural transition to making less estrogen. As your ovaries produce less estrogen, your periods become irregular. You may start to skip periods. Eventually, your monthly cycle will stop completely. Once you've gone a year without having a period, you've reached full menopause.

Symptoms in Perimenopause

Every woman's experience is unique. Some women have no symptoms or simply a few minor ones, while others experience a wide range of symptoms that can be quite severe. Symptoms begin in perimenopause but can continue into menopause. Fortunately, by the time you hit postmenopause, the major issues have all but vanished. Here is a look at the symptoms that begin in perimenopause and often persist into menopause:

Weight gain. This might be the symptom that brought you to this book! Whereas once you used to rip through nachos, candy bars, and cheeseburgers—and remain a size 4—now a few potato chips might force you into a larger dress size and elastic-waist pants become your new BFF.

When the pounds start inexplicably piling on, this is due mostly to the effects of changing hormones on appetite and metabolism, as well as those hormones that control how and where we store fat. This excess weight can increase and worsen other symptoms, such as night sweats and hot flashes, muscle and joint problems, and bladder issues.

The increase in hot flashes, in particular, has been chalked up to what researchers term the "thermoregulatory theory." If you carry more body fat on your frame relative to muscle, that body fat is insulating your body, making it harder to dissipate heat. Your body then retains that heat, and it can't be distributed. The result is more severe hot flashes.

Much of this has been substantiated in research. A 2017 study uncovered clear evidence that women who are overweight or obese have a more difficult menopause, with more night sweats and hot flashes. In addition, other symptoms like joint pain, muscle pain, vaginal dryness, and urinary incontinence and other bladder symptoms were worse in women with excess weight.

Another challenge for women in midlife has to do with visceral fat, which wraps around our organs. I call this the "menopause middle." It is caused by the rising activity of our circulating androgens (testosterone and others). Visceral fat is marked by an increasing waist-to-hip ratio (WHR). The WHR calculation is the ratio of your waist circumference to your hip circumference, and this gives a pretty fair indication of how much fat is stored on your waist, hips, and buttocks.

Aside from affecting the way we look (and how we feel about it), visceral fat is associated with increased risk for serious conditions like heart disease, breast cancer, uterine cancer, diabetes, hypertension, stroke, sleep apnea, and many other troubling diseases.

The point here is that if you can get your weight under control, you can go a long way toward easing many of the most severe symptoms of perimenopause and menopause—plus reduce your risk factors for many of these scary illnesses. Excess fat in midlife is not only a cosmetic concern but also an issue that can gravely affect health.

Hot flashes. You're all dressed up, you've done your hair, you've got your makeup on, when suddenly—wham. Here comes an intense heat whooshing through your upper torso and face. It might last anywhere from a few seconds to many minutes, but you're ready to strip down, right then and there. Some women have hot flashes once or twice a month, while others experience them daily. Nighttime hot flashes (night sweats) might wake you up, interrupt your sleep, and then make you feel weary and sluggish during the day.

Hair loss and changes. Your hair changes as you go through midlife. It usually thins out over parts of your scalp, as opposed to developing obvious bald patches. Also, your hair may fall out in big clumps when you brush or shower.

Hair loss during midlife is caused primarily by a hormonal imbalance that is specifically linked to the decline in estrogen, as well as the rise in the activity of testosterone. Hair grows more quickly and stays on your head longer when estrogen is abundant and testosterone activity is relatively low.

And where on Earth did those whiskers on your face and chin come from? Blame it also on the rising activity of testosterone.

Insomnia. Your sleep patterns may now resemble those of a newborn. You're up every two hours. You're hungry. And you have to pee. You toss and turn for hours each night, hoping that your mind will shut off and let you go to sleep.

You may be experiencing insomnia (difficulty falling asleep), or perhaps you wake up earlier than normal. Sweaty nights might also make it difficult to sleep.

Again, the culprit here is hormonal fluctuations. Your estrogen and progesterone levels are going up and down.

Memory loss and brain fog. You know that feeling when you're trying to remember something, and the word is right on the tip of your tongue? Or, you find yourself standing in the middle of the room and have no idea how you got there or what you're supposed to be doing? Or, you've repeated the same story to your husband or kids a couple of times already this week? This might be you 24/7 these days. This condition is often referred to as brain fog, and it's common during perimenopause and menopause because your body is producing less estrogen.

Vaginal and bladder problems. With the drop in estrogen levels, your vaginal walls become drier, thinner, and less elastic. I know one woman who described this dryness as feeling like her vagina had grown cobwebs! These changes may lead to pain and discomfort during intercourse. You may be more susceptible to vaginal infections when your estrogen levels are low.

Because of the proximity of the bladder to the vagina, the thinning of the vaginal wall affects the bladder, too. A loss of tissue tone may cause urinary incontinence and frequent bladder infections.

Sexual changes. Our sex lives—like life itself—are changeable based on many different situations. One such situation is the dip in female hormones during midlife. This change has many ramifications, including a decrease in sexual arousal and desire. However, if you were sexually frisky before menopause, you'll probably continue to have a healthy sex drive now. And if you wonder about sex after age 50 or 60 or beyond, the most important thing to remember is your sex life can and will last a lifetime—if you want it to!

Mood shifts. Irritable doesn't begin to describe it, right? Your emotions frequently spiral out of control at the least little thing, and you can't seem to control your mood swings and temper. Couple this with being tired (because you were woken up by hot flashes) and the problems are compounded. For many women, this is the worst symptom simply because you suddenly feel so *not like yourself.*

Yet again, one big reason for this change is your estrogen level. Estrogen controls how much serotonin is being produced in your brain. Serotonin is a chemical that helps regulate your moods. If you're producing less estrogen, you're also producing less serotonin. This can have a direct impact on how stable and optimistic you feel.

If you're dealing with mood shifts, remember that your body is changing and you aren't to blame for these emotions. It's also important that you explain the physiology of this particular symptom to your partner so that he or she can be more patient and understanding of, well, your impatience!

Other symptoms. Many other symptoms crop up during perimenopause, and very seldom are you warned about them. For example:

Breast pain
Dry and/or itchy skin
Palpitations
Panic attacks
Constipation
Dizziness
Dry mouth
Urinary incontinence
Rage
High blood pressure
High cholesterol
Dry eyes
Light-headedness
Headaches or migraines

The food and lifestyle strategies of the Galveston Diet will help you combat weight gain and other symptoms during perimenopause.

Menopause

After perimenopause comes menopause—the stage during which your ovaries stop producing reproductive hormones and you have no monthly periods for 12 consecutive months. Although the average age for starting menopause is 51, it is normal to experience it as early as 45 and as late as 55.

In menopause, weight gain can become even more pronounced—and frustrating to shed. On average, women gain between 12 and 15 pounds during the ages of 45 through 55. You'll experience more intense hunger signals, too, which make you want to eat more food and which necessarily increase your chances of putting on pounds.

What's more, other metabolic problems crop up at this time, including insulin resistance and disturbances in metabolizing glucose and fats. The risk of developing type 2 diabetes, osteoporosis, heart disease, and cancer increases, too.

An important study looked into how diet affects women when they enter menopause. It tracked 35,000 women for four years, and the results were astounding. Those whose diets were high in processed carbs, such as rice, pasta, potato chips, and pretzels, experienced menopause $1^1/_2$ years sooner, on average, than those women whose diet mainly consisted of fish and vitamin-rich foods (leafy vegetables, fruits, eggs, and so forth).

Why did women with the high intake of processed carbs hit menopause earlier? The researchers speculated that the high carbs spiked levels of circulating insulin, which probably caused insulin resistance and interfered with sex hormone activity.

The findings of this study give fair warning: Developing and maintaining healthy eating patterns sooner rather than later is critical to your health and menopause experience in midlife. That's what you're going to do on the Galveston Diet!

Unfortunately, a number of other health risks are associated with menopause, too. Before menopause, the estrogen generated by the ovaries protected us from heart attacks and strokes. Women lose a lot of this protection after menopause because less estrogen is produced. Midlife also brings other risk factors for heart disease, such as excessive cholesterol, high blood pressure, and a lack of physical activity.

You'll learn how to ease, manage, and even stop these symptoms once you're well into the Galveston Diet program.

The Joy of Change

Sandra had been overweight by 40 to 50 pounds her entire life. When she turned 50, she decided it was time to get healthy.

Frustrated by her lifelong struggle with her weight, Sandra fully embraced the Galveston Diet. She told us, "I could not believe the changes I've experienced."

Sandra lost 55 pounds and got down to a fit 120 pounds for the first time ever. Not only is the Galveston Diet effective for weight loss, but it also eases the symptoms of menopause. In Sandra's case, she found she was sleeping better and feeling more energized than she had in 20 years. She also no longer suffered back pain.

"I feel amazing!"

Postmenopause

Postmenopause is the stage of life after you have not had a period for 12 months or longer. During this stage, your cells may store even more fat and are slower to release it. Postmenopausal women have an almost five times higher risk of developing visceral fat, compared to premenopausal women.

Also, you may have less muscle mass, which makes your metabolism slow down, and your body doesn't burn calories as efficiently as it once did. Once you are postmenopausal, your hormone levels will remain at a constant low level.

I must point out that there are several health complications associated with postmenopause. To stay healthy in this phase of life, understand these conditions and their risk factors. That way, you can engage in ways, including good nutrition, to reduce your risk.

Osteoporosis. This is a medical issue that causes the thinning of your bones and makes you susceptible to bone fractures, particularly in the hips, spine, and wrists. Losses in bone density increase following menopause. You may lose up to 25 percent of your bone density up to age 60. This occurs because the amount of estrogen is declining in your body.

Osteoporosis affects one of every three postmenopausal women, and their remaining lifetime risk of fragility fractures is greater than the risk of developing breast cancer.

Even if you have been diagnosed with osteoporosis, you are not powerless. There are many treatments for it, and one of the best is to do weight-bearing exercises like resistance training. I love weight training. Not only does it make the muscles fit, but it also strengthens the bones. Your bones need to be resisting the force of gravity for the exercise to help in the prevention of further bone loss. Nutrition is key, too, and the Galveston Diet gives you what you need.

Cardiovascular disease. One of the biggest medical myths is that cardiovascular disease is a man's disease. It's the number one health threat for American women, especially during menopause and in postmenopause.

Menopause doesn't directly *cause* cardiovascular disease, but it may increase your risk of developing it. When the level of your hormones declines, the risk factors for heart trouble increase. You may develop high blood pressure, elevated LDL cholesterol (the unhealthy type), and a rise in triglycerides following menopause. According to the American Heart Association, one in three women will develop cardiovascular disease during menopause. There's also an increase in the incidence of heart attacks for women 10 years after menopause.

The Joy of Change

The Galveston Diet has been known to help women with high blood pressure. On the program, some people can even reduce their medication use (with permission from their physicians). Lesia is one of those people. Her medication was cut in half, which allowed her to maintain the same or better control of her blood pressure.

This situation often occurs with weight loss, especially with a reduction in visceral fat—which is what happened to Lesia. She lost several inches around her waist and is now wearing a single-digit pant size.

Depression and other mental health conditions. In postmenopause, the risk of developing depression appears to be greater than it is earlier in life. This most likely is due not only to a hormonal decline but also to major life changes during the postmenopausal years that can bring on depression, such as having the children leave home, the divorce or death of a spouse, stressful retirement planning, age-related health problems, and so forth.

A 2019 study looked into the frequency of depression in 371 premenopausal and postmenopausal women who were not on hormone replacement therapy. Just 21 percent of the premenopausal group experienced only mild depression, whereas nearly 60 percent of the postmenopausal women were suffering major depression (which is more dangerous than mild depression and requires urgent medical care).

If you're depressed, you may feel sad, irritable, and unmotivated, or sense you have bleak prospects for the future. You may feel like you're dragging yourself through the day. Normal, day-to-day activities may take longer and give you no satisfaction. Changes like these in your mental health should always be discussed with your doctor. Depression is highly treatable, and you do not have to live with it.

More severe vaginal dryness. Vaginal dryness typically begins in perimenopause, continues through menopause, and can become more severe in postmenopause. The vaginal walls shrink and thin as you get older, due to changes in hormone production. As the estrogen levels drop, less moisture is secreted by cells with thinner walls. This can lead to painful intercourse, frequent urinary tract infections (UTIs) or vaginal infections, and worsening incontinence.

There's no need to experience a sexual drought because of vaginal issues, including dryness. I'm a big believer in using a vaginal lubricant, and plenty of it. Many over-the-counter lubricants can be used to relieve dryness and pain in the vaginal region. They work by affecting the pH of the vaginal area, which also lowers the risk of a UTI. Be sure to select a lubricant designed exclusively for vaginal use. Avoid products with perfumes, herbal extracts, and artificial colors. (My favorite brands of lubricants are Uberlube and KY Silk-E.) Start using a lubricant well before you hit this stage of life, however, and you can keep feeling sensual and sexy—and make sex even more fun and intimate.

Also, consider talking to your doctor about a prescription for estrogen treatment in the form of a cream or ring that releases estrogen directly into the tissues in order to increase vaginal moisture.

The nutrition and lifestyle strategies you'll learn on the Galveston Diet will go a long way toward making your postmenopause years healthier and more satisfying.

Where Are You on Your Journey?

If you aren't sure where you are along your hormonal journey, take the short quiz that follows. It will measure the intensity of common symptoms and help you determine whether you are perimenopausal, menopausal, or postmenopausal—or not quite in one clear phase yet. You can then refer to your score when visiting your own doctor and use it as you follow the Galveston Diet.

Instructions: Rate the symptoms that follow, based on the severity with which you experience them. Circle either None, Mild, Moderate, or Severe.

1. Hot Flashes

- None
- Mild
- Moderate
- Severe

2. Light-Headed Feelings

- None
- Mild
- Moderate
- Severe

3. Headaches

- None
- Mild
- Moderate
- Severe

4. Irritability

- None
- Mild
- Moderate
- Severe

5. Depression

- None
- Mild
- Moderate
- Severe

6. Unloved Feelings

- None
- Mild
- Moderate
- Severe

7. Anxiety/Mood Changes

- None
- Mild
- Moderate
- Severe

8. Sleeplessness

- None
- Mild
- Moderate
- Severe

9. Unusual Tiredness

- None
- Mild
- Moderate
- Severe

10. Backache

- None
- Mild
- Moderate
- Severe

11. Joint Pains

- None
- Mild
- Moderate
- Severe

12. Muscle Pains

- None
- Mild
- Moderate
- Severe

13. New Facial Hair

- None
- Mild
- Moderate
- Severe

14. Dry Skin

- None
- Mild
- Moderate
- Severe

15. Crawling Feelings Under the Skin

- None
- Mild
- Moderate
- Severe

16. Low Libido/Fewer Sexual Feelings

- None
- Mild
- Moderate
- Severe

17. Uncomfortable Intercourse

- None
- Mild
- Moderate
- Severe

18. Dry Vagina

- None
- Mild
- Moderate
- Severe

19. Urinary Frequency

- None
- Mild
- Moderate
- Severe

20. Forgetfulness and/or Fuzzy Thinking (Brain Fog)

- None
- Mild
- Moderate
- Severe

Scoring: Review your answers and assign the following scores to each category: 0 for every None; 1 for every Mild; 2 for every Moderate; and 3 for every Severe.

Add up your score:

0–20: It is unlikely that your symptoms are related to perimenopause or menopause, although you may be starting to experience some symptoms.

21–40: It is possible that your symptoms are related to perimenopause or menopause.

41+: It is likely that your symptoms are related to perimenopause or menopause.

Three Strategies for Turning Things Around— The Galveston Diet

Not only have I personally gone through the physiological changes associated with perimenopause and menopause myself, but I have also ushered roughly 100,000 women through the Galveston Diet online program. All these experiences have helped me identify the secrets of combating the seemingly inevitable, stubborn fat, including belly fat, plus ways to resolve the health issues that plague women going through midlife.

Let's recap the three key actions involved in the Galveston Diet—strategies that you'll initiate in your own life very soon.

1. Intermittent Fasting

As I noted in the Introduction, intermittent fasting is key to the diet, especially during menopause. Even though it may seem intimidating, I promise you it's the easiest habit to develop and maintain!!

What is intermittent fasting? It is simply fasting for approximately 16 hours a day (much of it overnight) and then eating within a consecutive

8-hour window. It has a long list of benefits for women in midlife, and I cover this strategy in detail in Chapter 4.

2. Anti-Inflammatory Nutrition

Most of the time, inflammation in the body is a lifesaver. It empowers the body to fight off various disease-causing bacteria, viruses, and other pathogens. But sometimes, the whole feverish process doesn't shut down on cue, thereby having all sorts of health repercussions. For example, inflammation in the body can cause weight gain and make it hard for you to lose weight.

Fortunately, the Galveston Diet eases all this by cutting out foods that promote inflammation and encouraging foods that fight it. Added and simple sugars, as well as processed carbohydrates, are extremely inflammatory. Not to be dramatic, but at all costs, limit your consumption of these foods. It's even better for your health, your symptoms, and your weight to eliminate them altogether. Not only will doing so decrease the severity of menopausal symptoms but it will also reduce the frequency of them. That's a win-win right there!

More on this in Chapter 5.

3. Fuel Refocus

If you're otherwise healthy and eating a carbohydrate-centric diet, your body burns those calories for energy and stores any excess as fat. But to prevent fat storage and stimulate fat-burning, you must deplete the carbs. During the Fuel Refocus phase of the Galveston Diet, you'll adjust the ratios of macronutrients (protein, complex carbohydrates, and healthy fat) so as to encourage your body to utilize fat for fuel. Your new ratio will be 70 percent healthy fats, 20 percent lean protein, and 10 percent carbohydrates.

Refocusing your fuel like this does not mean you're following a keto diet. Traditional keto diets are extremely inflammatory for most people—which is why the Galveston Diet is not a keto diet. It focuses on lowering inflammation rather than promoting it.

The major caveat here is something delved into in Chapter 7: how to be picky with your carbohydrates. Choose those that are packed with fiber, vitamins, and antioxidants: quinoa, oats, sweet potatoes, blueberries, and apples are great examples of anti-inflammatory carbs.

When you start the Galveston Diet for Life program—which is a maintenance plan—you again change your macronutrient ratios to allow more carbohydrates and less fat. Ultimately, you'll refocus your macros to 40 percent fat, 20 percent protein, and 40 percent carbohydrates—and stabilize there.

The Joy of Change

When Paula came to the Galveston Diet, she was a desperate woman, having struggled with her weight since high school, suffering from polycystic ovary syndrome (PCOS) in her twenties, and surviving thyroid cancer in her thirties.

Nothing she tried had helped her drop pounds, and by her forties, she was gaining even more weight. She had just about given up. Paula is a firefighter who knows the importance of being healthy and staying in shape—but all this had eluded her until she started the Galveston Diet.

She said this about her experience: "I started intermittent fasting, eating anti-inflammatory foods, and counting my macros in order to refocus my fuel. The weight just started falling off. It seemed too easy! My endocrinologist cut my metformin for PCOS in half and thinks I can go off it completely. I truly believe this diet has healed the insulin resistance I've struggled with for over 20 years. I believe it prevented a diagnosis of type 2 diabetes."

Support from friends and loved ones is so important when

you're changing your lifestyle. Paula's husband followed the program right along with her and lost 50 pounds himself.

She added, "I can't tell you how this has changed our lives. It is definitely a way of life for us now."

Hot Flash: Don't Neglect Regular Exercise

As part of the Galveston Diet lifestyle, I strongly encourage a mix of strength training and regular cardio (fast walking, jogging, cardio machines—whatever you enjoy). Don't be afraid of weights! Even light ones help. Our muscles naturally shrink a bit through an aging process called sarcopenia. If we're not doing weight-bearing exercise, we lose muscle mass, and this slows down our metabolism. The net effect—you guessed it—is unexplained weight gain! Also, performing cardio and weight-bearing exercises will keep you burning calories for longer after your workout, so that's another win-win.

Move Forward with the Right Attitude

Throughout our lives, we women pass through beautiful gateways. Getting our period is the gateway to womanhood; for some, becoming pregnant and then having children is the gateway to motherhood. Both are seen as miraculous wins, while menopause is commonly described as a loss—a loss of fertility, of beauty, of sexuality, and of self-worth.

But I would argue that menopause is the gateway to a new life that carries a large upside. Forty percent of a woman's life is spent in postmenopause. Let that sink in for a moment.

Imagine what you can do with all that time! Menopause tends to coincide with a time when your children—if you have them—are launching or have launched adult lives of their own. This means you have more time for yourself, with an opportunity to reimagine your future life. You have time to uncover and embrace your passions—start a new business, devote your energies to a cause, write, pursue art, spend more time with family and friends, enjoy nature, run for office, or follow whatever interest matters to you. Anything!

Along those lines, consider menopause to be a privilege. It means you've lived a long time—an opportunity many others don't enjoy, for one reason or another. For example, I celebrate my birthday in a big way each year because I'm so grateful to be here—even if that means a few wrinkles, some gray hair, and creaky joints.

So, view this period as a time to learn more about yourself. Instead of feeling bad about this phase of life and being upset with the symptoms, be intentional about your choices. Learn more about your body and what does and doesn't work for you, whether it's food, exercise, or relationships—and then focus on the positives rather than the negatives. If you can reframe the way you think about menopause, and you live the principles in the Galveston Diet, this can be an amazing time in your life.

CHAPTER 2

Getting a Handle on Your Hormones

For far too long, we've been fed the lie that losing weight and keeping it off is simply a matter of willpower. Grit your teeth, white knuckle it, and off go the pounds. But if you "fall off the diet wagon," you're a failure.

Here's the truth: you're not a failure. You didn't fail any of the diets you tried; those diets failed you. Your past issues with losing weight and keeping it off *are not your fault.* And they have very little to do with willpower.

The real issue is hormones. Hormones and metabolic factors connected to them are the reason we tend to put on pounds during midlife.

When you have trouble losing weight, you feel frustrated and powerless, sometimes beating yourself up for failing at dieting. This creates a vicious cycle of weight loss and weight gain, with lots of unnecessary emotional pressure involved. But weight gain has nothing to do with you, your moral character, or your personality. Repeat after me: it's hormones!

The Flawed Science of Weight Gain

For nearly a century, the cause of weight gain and obesity has been described as "an energy imbalance between calories consumed and calories expended," to quote the World Health Organization. In other words, obesity is an energy-balance disorder: calories in minus calories out = fat loss. I believed this, too. It was what I was taught in medical school and residency. As it turns out, this line of thinking has been proven by modern obesity research to be largely inadequate.

Fortunately, this entire paradigm is now being challenged. A major study published in 2020 in the *American Journal of Clinical Nutrition* and authored by many of the leading scientists in obesity clearly points out that obesity is *not* an energy-balance disorder but, rather, a hormonal disorder that dictates fat storage and metabolism regardless of how many calories you eat.

In plain language, your weight is controlled largely by hormones, which in turn are influenced dramatically by the *quality* of the nutrition you consume (particularly carbohydrates) and less by the *quantity* of the food you eat. You don't only put on weight because you eat too much or take in more calories than you burn. You also gain weight because the carbohydrates in your diet—both the quantity of carbs and their quality—establish a hormonal environment that makes you pile on fat pounds. Plus, as women, we deal with declining estrogen levels as we get older, and we find new fat accumulating around our waistlines—no matter how much rabbit food we eat or treadmill miles we log!

The Joy of Change

All her life, Steph had a terrible time losing weight, and every attempt had failed spectacularly. Trying to rely on willpower, she followed low-fat, food pyramids, calorie counting, carb lovers—you name the diet, she did it.

Even more scary, her weight had contributed to some serious

health issues. Five years ago, she was diagnosed as pre-diabetic and hypertensive. Both conditions could worsen if she did not make lifestyle changes.

Steph was prompted into action, fortunately, after looking at some family vacation photos on her phone. She did not like her overweight appearance; in fact, she was shocked at how much weight she had put on.

Steph found out about the Galveston Diet—and was intrigued. It bore no resemblance to anything she had tried. It was geared to regulating hormonal weight gain by nutritionally shifting your fuel sources away from too many carbs and inflammatory foods.

Steph began following the Galveston Diet—and met with great success.

"I am down over 60 pounds in eight months. It has not only helped me lose the weight I so desperately needed to lose, but I am no longer pre-diabetic, and I am no longer on blood pressure medication. I feel better than I have in over 20 years."

You and Your Hormones

Hormones are your body's chemical messengers. Dozens of glands and organs—including the gut, ovaries, adrenal glands, and brain—are pumping out various hormones all the time. They act on cells throughout the body, telling them how to behave. And they're constantly chatting with one another and other compounds in the body to stay in balance.

When it comes to your weight and other perimenopause and menopause symptoms, hormones are running the show. They control appetite, hunger, food cravings, metabolic rate, fat gain and distribution, and hunger, among other things. If certain hormones are out of whack, your weight-loss efforts can be sabotaged. What's more, and as outlined in Chapter 1, suboptimal levels of certain hormones are linked not only to obesity but also to chronic inflammation, heart disease, stroke, diabetes, and more.

Fortunately, regulating your hormones helps prevent weight gain and fights inflammation. The power to do all this is in your hands—with the nutritionally based strategies you'll learn in *The Galveston Diet.*

The key to resolving hormonal weight gain and other midlife symptoms comes down to nine hormones—and managing them primarily through nutrition.

Estrogen

Estrogen is the primary female sex hormone most closely associated with perimenopause and menopause. *Estrogen* is an umbrella term for three chemically similar hormones: estrone, estradiol, and estriol. Their main job is to orchestrate the expression of female sex characteristics and to regulate the menstrual cycle. Estrogen also allows body fat to be distributed on the thighs, buttocks, and abdomen. During your reproductive years, additional fat deposited in these locations provides an energy source for eventual pregnancy and lactation.

This hormone affects your health in many other ways, too. For example:

- It helps build your bones and maintain bone strength.
- It helps control cholesterol levels.
- It increases blood supply to the skin and regulates the thickness of the skin.
- It keeps the pelvic floor and vaginal and bladder tissues strong and healthy.
- It helps even out your moods and may manage anxiety and depression.

As we enter midlife, our estrogen begins to fluctuate greatly. When the ovaries begin to decrease the production of estrogen in perimenopause, the body ramps up the production of follicular stimulating hormone (FSH) to try to get the ovaries to produce more estrogen. This leads to some of the wild fluctuations of estrogen during perimenopause.

As estrogen levels decline during the transition to menopause, the liver begins to decrease the production of sex hormone-binding globulin (SHBG). SHBG binds our sex hormones and renders them inactive. As SHBG levels drop, the activity of our sex hormones, particularly androgens (like testosterone), increases. This chain of hormonal events leads to changes in cholesterol, visceral fat gain, and unwanted hair growth.

How the Galveston Diet Helps Manage Estrogen

When you get to the food recommendations in Chapter 7, you'll see a heavy focus on cruciferous and green vegetables, as well as on avocados, salmon, and seeds. All these foods help offset the effects of your fluctuating estrogen. Here's how:

Cruciferous vegetables, like broccoli, broccoli sprouts, Brussels sprouts, and cauliflower, are tightly linked to estrogen. Research shows that women who eat a diet rich in cruciferous vegetables have a lower risk of heart disease, stroke, and cancer, and overall better hormone and estrogen levels.

One of the problems experienced by many women in midlife is that they have excess estrogen in their bodies, rather than too little. If this has happened to you, your body is not ovulating regularly, leading to unopposed estrogen production and little to no progesterone production. Or your body is not breaking down estrogen and removing it from your body as it should. Having excess body fat can also lead to high estrogen levels, as androgens are converted to estrogen in our fat cells.

Other causes include drinking too much alcohol; having liver problems, in which your body cannot properly metabolize estrogen; or being overexposed to synthetic "xenoestrogens," which are chemicals found in the environment that act like estrogen once they're inside your body. The latter can increase your estrogen levels.

One of the ways to combat high estrogen is to eat more cruciferous vegetables. These vegetables contain a phytochemical called diindolylmethane (DIM) that helps rid the body of *excess* estrogen. Cruciferous vegetables also contain sulfur compounds that help detoxify a sluggish liver, which can trigger weight gain, bloating, gas, and constipation.

Leafy greens also contain DIM, as well as chemicals such as indole-3-carbinol (I3C) and calcium D-glucarate, all of which help increase the liver's ability to clear estrogen metabolites (these are the by-products of estrogen metabolism) from the body.

Avocados are packed with healthy fats, which are associated with balancing progesterone and estrogen.

Fish high in omega-3 fatty acids can help support estrogen production. Salmon in particular contains optimal amounts of omega-3 fatty acids.

Flax seeds and pumpkin seeds contain dietary lignans that help inhibit enzymes involved in healthy estrogen metabolism. Lignans are plant nutrients that are high in fiber. They also serve as antioxidants that support your immune system. What's more, lignans are excellent for managing hormone levels in the body, particularly estrogen.

Pumpkin seeds are rich in zinc, essential fats, and protein, making them one of the best foods to help balance estrogen.

Insulin

Insulin is a hormone produced by your pancreas in response to how many carbohydrates you eat. It has many functions, but insulin's main job is to allow your cells to take in sugar from your blood and store it for energy (depending on what is needed).

Another of insulin's vital roles in the body relates to fat storage. It obstructs the breakdown of fat tissue and stimulates the creation of body fat. So, if you are overweight, diabetic, or predisposed to diabetes, you must normalize your insulin levels as much as possible to prevent fat storage and to manage your weight. An important solution is to restrict your intake of carbohydrates, especially refined carbs and added sugar.

As we age and develop more visceral fat (belly fat), insulin resistance (IR) can develop, meaning it takes more insulin than normal to "push" sugar into the cells to do their job.

A diet rich in sugar, refined carbohydrates, and fast food drives insulin resistance and therefore weight gain. One fascinating study found that people who ate at fast-food restaurants habitually—twice a week or more—gained weight and developed insulin resistance, suggesting that fast food increases the risk of obesity and type 2 diabetes.

Hot Flash: Signs You May Be Insulin Resistant

- You have extreme thirst or hunger.
- You feel hungry even after a meal.
- You experience frequent vaginal or bladder infections.
- You have increased abdominal circumference and body fat.
- You have to pee more often.
- You get tingling in your hands and feet.
- You're getting skin tags.
- You have dark, velvet patches on your neck and armpits—a skin condition known as acanthosis nigricans.

How the Galveston Diet Helps Normalize Insulin Levels and Improve Insulin Sensitivity

On the Galveston Diet, you'll be changing your eating habits to naturally manage your insulin levels and restore them to normal. Here's what we'll concentrate on:

Limiting carbohydrates. Lower-carb diets have been proven to reduce insulin levels and stabilize blood sugar levels. You'll learn how to manage your carbohydrates in the Fuel Refocus phase of the Galveston Diet.

Cutting back on or avoiding added or processed sugars. High amounts of dietary fructose, in the form of high-fructose corn syrup and sucrose, promote insulin resistance and raise insulin levels.

Enjoying ample protein at meals. Although insulin levels rise initially after eating protein, the long-term effects of eating protein lead to decreases in belly fat and, therefore, help prevent IR.

Serving up healthy fats. Foods rich in omega-3 fats, in particular, have been found to help lower fasting insulin levels.

Boosting your fiber. It's important to keep track of your total fiber intake and ensure you are getting at least 25 grams daily (I shoot for 35 grams per day). It's also important to obtain a combination of soluble and insoluble fiber. Soluble fiber dissolves in water, forming a gel-like substance that helps slow down digestion and the absorption of sugars. Examples of soluble fiber–rich foods include lentils, nuts, oats, and certain fruits and vegetables.

Insoluble fiber does not dissolve in water, but it helps food move through the digestive system more quickly. Examples of foods containing insoluble fiber include vegetables and whole grains. As the name suggests, insoluble fiber does not dissolve in water, which gives it the ability to remain fully intact in the digestive tract. This allows it to add bulk to the stool and thus have a laxative effect that can be used to treat digestive issues like constipation.

Supplementing with magnesium. Insulin-resistant people are often deficient in magnesium, so supplementing with this mineral can improve insulin sensitivity. We'll get into greater detail about importance of magnesium in your diet in Chapter 7.

Eating antioxidant-rich foods. Colorful fruits and vegetables contain antioxidants that fight inflammation and lead to lower insulin levels.

Flavoring foods with spices and herbs. I try to use various spices and herbs in almost all my recipes. Some of the best flavorings I've found include fenugreek (full of soluble fiber), turmeric (a powerful antioxidant and inflammation fighter), ginger (improves the function of glucose receptors on muscle cells), garlic (another powerful antioxidant), and cinnamon (1 to 6 grams or $^1/_4$ to $1^1/_2$ teaspoons daily for regulating blood sugar).

Sipping green tea. Green tea is high in antioxidants that help fight inflammation and increase insulin sensitivity.

Getting consistent exercise. Regular cardio exercise and resistance training improve insulin sensitivity.

Leptin

Produced by fat cells, leptin is known as the "I'm full," or the satiety, hormone. It reduces the appetite and makes you feel full after eating. What's more, leptin tells your brain that there's enough fat in storage and that no more is needed, which helps prevent overeating.

Ironically, when you're overweight, you probably have too much leptin in your bloodstream—so much so that your body doesn't register the "I'm full" sensation. In fact, one study found that leptin levels in obese people were four times higher than in people of a healthy weight.

A lack of sensitivity to leptin leads to a condition known as leptin resistance. With leptin resistance, the brain can't recognize leptin signals and thus it drives cravings, unhealthy eating habits, and weight gain. A vicious cycle can ensue. You eat more and put on body fat. More body fat creates more leptin in the fat cells and elevates insulin levels. Excess body fat disrupts the proper leptin signaling and thus worsens insulin resistance. In essence, your brain thinks you're starving, which makes you want to eat more. You put on even more weight and yet feel hungrier, so you eat more and gain even more fat. And on and on.

Hot Flash: Nix These Six Foods to Prevent Leptin Resistance

Gaining visceral fat (belly fat) and eating a lot of high-fructose corn syrup in processed foods are the two biggest reasons you might be leptin resistant. To solve this problem and avoid leptin resistance, get rid of the following foods in your diet:

- Soft drinks
- Sweetened fruit juices
- Canned fruits
- Boxed desserts
- Flavored yogurt
- Sugary breakfast cereals

How the Galveston Diet Helps Manage Leptin

Paying attention to your eating habits is critical for managing leptin, and it's actually easier than you think. Here's how you can do that on the Galveston Diet:

Avoid processed food. These foods may drive inflammation, which causes leptin resistance.

Eat more fiber. It helps control your appetite, satiety, and weight. Soluble fiber, in particular, can help improve your gut health.

Lower your triglycerides. This is the most common form of fat in the bloodstream. Having high triglycerides can halt the transportation of leptin from your blood to your brain, preventing the leptin's fullness signal from reaching your brain. The brain then thinks you're starving and initiates powerful mechanisms to make your body regain that lost fat. The best way to lower triglycerides is to reduce your carbohydrate intake.

Focus on protein. Eating adequate protein can support weight loss, resulting from an improvement in leptin sensitivity. As a woman, if you're eating three times a day, you should have at least 20 to 25 grams of protein per meal. Every ounce of animal protein (which includes everything from fish and poultry to pork and steak) contains about 8 grams of protein, while vegetarian sources of protein like hard-boiled eggs and a half a cup of beans have about 8 and 11 grams, respectively. Serving up a 3-ounce portion of quality protein three times a day is one of the easiest ways to hit your protein quota.

Exercise regularly. Physical activity may help reverse leptin resistance.

Improve your sleep quality. Poor sleep is implicated in problems with leptin.

Ghrelin

Ghrelin is a hormone made in your gut. It travels through your bloodstream to your brain, where it signals your brain to seek out food and eat. Thus, its main function is to increase your appetite.

If you severely restrict your calories, the ghrelin levels will shoot up, and you're likely to feel ravenous—which is one reason why cutting calories makes it so hard to stick to a diet.

How the Galveston Diet Helps Improve the Function of Ghrelin

The more ghrelin that's secreted, the hungrier you are and the more you want to eat, so it's easy to see why you want to keep your ghrelin levels under control! Here's how the Galveston Diet does that:

Ease back on sugar intake. Avoid added sugars, especially high-fructose corn syrup sweetened drinks.

Eat protein at every meal. This is especially the case when you break a fast. For a woman over 50, a great goal is approximately 20 to 25 grams or around 3 ounces at each meal.

Eat high-fiber foods at meals. Fiber fills you up quickly and increases satiety. It also prevents blood sugar levels from spiking after a meal.

Cortisol

As if midlife weren't hard enough just to get through, there's also stress—and plenty of it. We have stress at home, with our families, at work . . . stress, stress, stress. When you're under stress, your body releases stress hormones, and one of these is cortisol.

When you're faced with a stressor, cortisol stimulates the release of fat and carbohydrates to give you the energy to fight or flee the situation. This sudden energy surge can help you survive in a crisis or run away from danger. The problem is that cortisol doesn't know the difference between true emergencies (avoiding a collision or running from an assailant) and chronic "dangers" like financial worries, deadlines, family problems, and other challenges of a fast-paced lifestyle.

When stress is chronic and unresolved, a constant stream of cortisol floods your body. This may raise your blood sugar, alter your appetite, stimulate your cravings, increase the rate at which you store fat, and redistribute your fat to be stored viscerally. Chronically elevated cortisol can also cause cells to become resistant to insulin.

How the Galveston Diet Regulates Cortisol

If you've ever been through a time in your life when you were constantly stressed out, you probably felt less like yourself and more like a worn-out shell of yourself. Cortisol—higher levels of it than usual—is the culprit. That's why it's of utmost importance to figure out how to *lower* the cortisol. And you can do it with certain foods you'll find on the Galveston Diet:

Dark chocolate. After a hard day, some sweetness always seems to satisfy—which is why I reach for a little dark chocolate. With 70 percent or greater cocoa content, it has plenty of essential nutrients, for one thing. Plus, it's a stress reliever. Two studies of 95 adults showed that consuming dark chocolate reduced their cortisol response to a stress challenge.

Include probiotics and prebiotics in your diet. Probiotics are friendly, symbiotic bacteria in foods such as yogurt, sauerkraut, and kimchi. Various studies have shown that increases in the probiotics in the gut can curb inflammation and cortisol levels, and that this can help reduce symptoms of depression, anxiety, and stress.

Found in soluble fiber, prebiotics are food for these bacteria in the gut and have been found to help reduce cortisol levels.

Water your body. Staying well hydrated can keep physiological stress levels down. When you do not supply your body with ample fluids, you're putting stress on it, and it will respond by increasing the cortisol levels. How do you know if you are well hydrated? Look in the toilet. The color of your urine should be very light yellow to clear. Anything darker can indicate dehydration.

Focus on fish oil. Foods rich in omega-3 fatty acids have been shown to reduce cortisol. Don't confuse omega-3 fats with omega-6 fats! Omega-6 fatty acids—found in processed snacks, fast foods, cakes, fatty meats, and cured meats—tend to *promote* inflammation.

Lifestyle modifications also help regulate cortisol. As you're transitioning through the hormonal changes of midlife, these strategies are even more important:

Manage stress. There are lots of ways to relieve stress, from engaging in relaxation programs to those devoted to stress management, to yoga. One of the best strategies I've found is meditation. It has been shown to significantly reduce cortisol levels. Consider a trial subscription to the Calm or Headspace apps to give you a beginner's framework for meditation. Also, the simple act of listening to music you enjoy can reduce levels of stress-induced cortisol.

Strive for quality sleep. In several studies, people getting less sleep or poor quality sleep had significantly higher cortisol levels compared to control groups.

Work it out. Numerous studies have shown that moderate exercise decreases cortisol levels.

Neuropeptide Y

Many people talk about the addictive power of carbohydrates. I certainly agree—and the ease with which you can get hooked on them is something I've heard from many of my patients, too. But like weight gain, these addictive-like cravings are not your fault. Blame them on neuropeptide Y (NPY)! That's the hormone that drives carbohydrate cravings.

Another crazy aspect of NPY is that it is also highly involved in the motivation and search for food. Those times when you've rummaged through the fridge looking for food? That's NPY at work.

Produced by cells in the brain and nervous system, neuropeptide Y is one of the most powerful stimulators of appetite. It is triggered by low leptin levels and caloric restriction (which partly explains why so many diets fail); its levels are highest when we are fasting and lowest after a meal. Additionally, levels of NPY are elevated during times of stress, which can lead to overeating and visceral fat gain.

NPY tends to lead us to *decrease* the time between meals, makes us feel more motivated to eat, and delays the brain's signal that we are full.

How the Galveston Diet Lowers NPY

When you start refocusing your fuel on the Galveston Diet, you can expect your carb cravings to become a thing of the past. Here's how to make this a habit:

Eat the right amount of protein. People on low-protein diets can often have elevated NPY levels. Adequate protein for a woman over 50 is 20 to 25 grams, or about 3 ounces of high-quality protein, three times a day.

Include enough prebiotic soluble fiber in your diet. Soluble fiber feeds the friendly bacteria in the digestive system to ensure a healthy gut and fights cravings for carbs when you don't need them.

Manage stress. Similar to cortisol, NPY can be lowered by adopting behaviors that decrease stress in your life.

Glucagon-Like Peptide-1

A hormone made by your gut when nutrients enter the intestines is glucagon-like peptide 1 (GLP-1). Higher levels of GLP-1 curb your appetite and are linked to weight loss. This hormone also slows down the digestion process and helps nutrients be released more evenly. It improves insulin production in the body and prevents your liver from releasing more sugar into your blood than needed. GLP-1 is thus very important to blood sugar and insulin control.

How the Galveston Diet Increases GLP-1

When you start following the Galveston Diet, you'll find yourself increasingly less hungry, with fewer cravings. One big reason is that you'll be eating more foods that boost GLP-1. My recommendations are as follows:

Fish, whey protein (cottage cheese, ricotta cheese, and milk), and yogurt. These foods have been shown to increase GLP-1 levels and improve insulin sensitivity. (Whey is the watery milk that has separated from the curds when cheese is made.)

Foods rich in antioxidants (mainly vegetables and fruits). These foods prevent chronic inflammation, which is linked to lower GLP-1 levels, so a diet with these nutrients can increase GLP-1 levels. Also, leafy greens like spinach and kale have been shown in research to stimulate higher GLP-1 levels and support weight loss.

Probiotic foods, such as yogurt. Probiotics have been shown to increase GLP-1 levels and decrease food intake.

Cholecystokinin

Here is another very interesting hormone—cholecystokinin (CCK). It is beneficial to anyone who wants to lose weight—for two main reasons.

First, it works like an appetite suppressant, curbing your food intake. This is definitely an advantage if you're trying to eat less and shed body fat. This is the case because the CCK slows down the rate at which food moves through your digestive tract, giving you the sensation of feeling full longer.

Second, CCK stimulates the breakdown of fat tissue so it can be burned. This helps improve your body composition, as well as appetite control.

In the body, CCK is manufactured by specialized cells in the intestinal lining when you eat a meal that contains fat. Basically, it triggers the release of bile and pancreatic enzymes for fat digestion.

How the Galveston Diet Increases CCK

You'll be eating the following foods for lots of other reasons, too (see previous reasons!), but they also enhance CCK production: Eat foods rich in protein, fat, and fiber. Also, eat foods high in omega-3 fatty acids, such as fish.

Pancreatic Peptide YY

The pancreatic peptide YY (PYY) is a hormone produced in the small intestine. It is released after eating and it suppresses your appetite. In fact, it is one of the hormones that makes you feel full after eating because it slows the emptying of your stomach.

The amount of PYY dispatched into the blood depends on the type of food you eat. Fats and protein, for example, stimulate the greatest release of this hormone. Its secretion can also be stimulated by digestive juices (such as bile).

Levels of PYY are highest in the second hour after eating, after which they gradually decrease. Low levels of PPY are seen during long periods without eating, such as overnight.

With low PYY concentrations, you'll feel an increase in your appetite, and you'll want to keep eating. People who are obese or who have type 2 diabetes tend to have low levels—which obviously then aggravates weight gain.

How the Galveston Diet Increases PYY

The meal plans you follow on the Galveston Diet are geared to help you regulate PYY, along with other hormones. As you'll see, the ideal scenario is as follows:

Eat a lower-carb diet. This is done in an effort to stabilize blood glucose levels. Elevated blood sugar may hinder PYY's effects.

Eat sufficient amounts of protein. The protein can come from either animal or plant sources; my meal plans will show you how.

Include adequate fiber. Getting enough fiber is essential in your diet.

Understanding how hormones impact your weight and other symptoms is an important first step toward good health. When you realize that your behavior concerning food is hormonally driven, you can stop beating yourself up for supposed failures and concentrate on changing the pattern of your eating. You have far more control over your body than you realize! You have nothing to lose—except those stubborn pounds!

Hot Flash: Should You Consider Hormone Replacement Therapy?

Great progress has been made in the field of hormone replacement therapy (HRT), and it's here to stay. HRT can be life-changing for many women.

HRT has so many benefits. It can:

Whittle your waistline by reducing abdominal fat

Redistribute your body fat so that you're a little more proportional

Lower fasting glucose and insulin levels, helping to prevent insulin resistance and type 2 diabetes

Improve blood lipid profiles, including cholesterol and triglycerides, often the scourge of a healthy heart, and therefore cut your risk of cardiovascular disease

Reduce bone loss, thereby helping to prevent osteoporosis

Improve cognition (less brain fog!)

Enhance your sense of well-being

No one can decide if HRT is right for you except you and your doctor, but the more science-based information you have, the more informed your choice will be and the more confident you'll feel about your decision. Here are some of the key factors I discuss with women who are considering HRT:

- Generally, you should start treatment during perimenopause or in the first few years after menopause.
- Realize that it is mainly the deficiency of estrogen in your system that causes some of your weight gain and other noticeable symptoms of perimenopause and menopause. For this reason, HRT has been approved only to treat vasomotor disturbances (changes in the function of the vascular system such hot flashes) and to reverse vaginal changes, such as the thinning of the vaginal wall and lack of lubrication. The FDA has not approved HRT for losing visceral fat or reducing inflammation (although HRT can help with both).
- If you have a uterus, understand that you must not take estrogen alone, due to the risk of endometrial cancer. The

addition of progesterone to the therapy decreases this risk, and combination therapy is always the therapy of choice. If you do not have a uterus, progesterone is not necessary.

Please consult a physician who is knowledgeable about HRT and can individualize it to your particular situation. See Resources on page 261 for a link to a list of "menopause friendly" health care providers on my website.

CHAPTER 3

Prepare to Change Your Life

You know that losing weight and resolving midlife symptoms while you're on the Galveston Diet will make you healthier. The very good news is that once you're well into the program, you can substantially reduce belly fat, hot flashes, fatigue, brain fog, bad moods, and more. I've seen women just two weeks into the program begin to experience these positive changes. So every effort you make is going to be rewarded!

That said, I know you're eager to begin your new lifestyle. But before you actually jump in, I want to caution you to ease into the plan. Take at least a few days or a week to read through this book. It's important that you know exactly what is going on in your body at this stage of your life, that you understand why the program contains what it does, and that you see how the three components work together. You need to understand what the meal plans entail and why they are constructed as they are.

Let this information really sink in. When you arm yourself with nutritional knowledge, you will be more successful with the lifestyle changes and will make greater progress toward reducing disease risk and becoming healthier.

So, again, my first piece of advice is to not rush. Take time to invest in yourself. You have the rest of your life to master the plan! That said, here are several preparatory steps that will help you be successful.

Know Your Measurements

You won't know how very successful you've been unless you have a clear vision of where you started—where you are now. So, it's important to take certain bodily measurements and occasionally use your scale to gauge your results.

1. Check your beginning weight. I teach my students on the Galveston Diet to "break up" with their scale. I know this feels scary, so let's talk about it. The scale is helpful, but it's not the only measure there is, because it doesn't really assess how healthy you are. Remember, the main goal of this program is to get you as healthy as possible. It is common for women on this program to lose inches, especially around the waist, without any weight loss registering on the scale. This occurs because they are most likely gaining lean muscle while losing body fat, and muscle generally weighs more than fat. Plus, muscle takes up less space on the body. It's okay to consider the number on the scale in your overall assessment, but do not allow it to be the final word.

So, weigh yourself today, write down that weight in a little notebook along with the date, and keep that notebook handy. Just remember that your weight is only one data point to gauge your progress; don't get obsessed with what the scale says.

2. Take your body's circumference measurements. Buy a cloth tape measure and measure your hip, abdominal, and inner thigh circumferences. Write the measurements down in your notebook where you've recorded your weight measurement.

Here are some tips for measuring:

- For accuracy, take your measurements in the nude first thing in the morning, prior to breaking your fast, so as to avoid any post-meal bloating.
- Breathe normally and don't "suck in" to get a better number. You want your measurements to reflect your true stats.
- Measure yourself in front of a mirror to ensure that your tape measure is held straight.
- For your waist circumference, stand up straight and exhale. Measure around the smallest part of your waist; for many women, this is just above your navel, but yours might be higher.

Note: Your waist measurement is one of the most important assessments of your overall health. Too much fat around the waist indicates that you might be carrying excess visceral fat. Visceral fat presents significant health risks. Ideally, you should have a waist circumference of below 35 inches.

- For your hip circumference, measure the distance around the widest part of your buttocks. Although everyone varies, the hip measurement is about 7 inches below the waist.
- Pull the tape so that it is snug but not too tight.

3. Calculate your waist-to-hip ratio. Your waist-to-hip ratio (WHR) is the gauge of your body weight distribution, particularly in terms of health. In fact, it is the most important assessment you'll take on the Galveston Diet because it indicates how healthy you are, as well as pointing to any health risks you may be facing. As your WHR improves, your health will improve—which is the number one goal of this program.

Now, to calculate your WHR, divide your waist circumference by your hip circumference. Record the WHR and add it to your little notebook.

4. Take a photo of yourself. It may feel uncomfortable or daunting to

ust me, later on you will love being able to see your results as
ɛss through the program.

Following the plan, you will again measure yourself after four weeks and will recalculate your WHR. Expect to be totally inspired by the inches and pounds you've trimmed off your body—a sign that you're burning pure fat and improving your overall health.

Your WHR and Your Health

A very large body of scientific evidence shows that a high WHR can forecast cardiovascular disease, hypertension, diabetes, gallbladder disease, even cancer.

Menopausal women often see a significant increase in their WHR—which implies that they are at significant risk for heart disease, hip fracture, and certain cancers (including breast cancer and endometrial cancer). On a positive note, researchers have also found that decreasing your WHR is associated with greater health benefits and lowered risk of developing these diseases.

As a general guide, here's a commonly used chart to give you an idea of what your current waist-to-hip ratio might foreshadow.

Waist-to-Hip Ratio

Health Risk	Women
Low	0.80 or lower
Moderate	0.81–0.85
High	0.86 or higher

Get a Nutrition Tracker

Since founding the organization and creating the Galveston Diet in 2017, I've observed that the women who are the most successful with the program monitor their micronutrients and macronutrients (the "macros").

Macronutrients are the three categories of nutrients you eat the most and that provide you with most of your fuel: carbohydrates, protein, and fat. Micronutrients, on the other hand, are vital nutrients your body uses in smaller amounts: vitamins, minerals, fiber, antioxidants, and phytochemicals. You can track both of these via a phone app.

My favorite nutrition tracking app is Cronometer. This app has a comprehensive and extensive nutritional database that helps you develop the habit of refocusing your fuel. Other good tracker apps are Carb Manager, MyFitnessPal, Fitbit, Lose It!, and MyNetDiary. You'll need a smartphone, of course. After downloading the app of choice, you use the database to start gaining control of your nutrition choices and become more mindful of your intake. Using these apps is akin to using cash or a debit card rather than a credit card to pay for something; you always know exactly where you are in your nutritional "budget."

It's a good idea to make sure the app you choose can track customized macro percentages and net carbs (total carbs minus fiber; see page 106 for more on why this is important). As an experiment, use your chosen app to start keeping track of what you eat this initial week.

Of course, you won't be tracking or counting calories on the Galveston Diet. As mentioned earlier, counting calories isn't the best approach to weight loss—and here's why. Calories are not created equal; different foods have vastly different effects on your hormones, energy expenditures, and feelings of hunger. When you eat low-quality, processed foods that are high in empty calories, your body never feels satisfied. It continues to ask you for more food, in the hope you'll keep feeding it and supply more nutrients. Translation: you overeat and you gain weight.

The opposite happens when you enjoy high-quality, nutritious foods. You're less likely to overeat because you're nourishing your body with what it needs, in the appropriate amounts. For most people, simply changing their food selections to those on this plan will support weight loss, burn fat, discourage cravings, and build health.

Start a Daily Journaling Practice

I'm a strong believer in daily journaling. The practice of sitting down and recording your thoughts each day helps you focus on setting and achieving your goals (mental, physical, dietary, activity, and so forth). Such contemplation also leads to practicing gratitude for help or encouragement you've received from others. Journaling is essentially a way to hold yourself accountable. Your journal is also a great place to document your body measurements and WHR. You can also use the first couple pages of your journal to record your personal health and weight goals.

The amount of journaling you choose to do is individual, and by all means feel free to write about whatever is on your mind. But in terms of the program, here are some topics to consider each day:

Today I am grateful for:________________________________

Two self-care practices I will do just for me:________________

Today's victories or celebrations:_________________________

My daily intentions:___________________________________

(Note: These are personal commitments, such as "I will try something challenging today," "I accept myself as enough," "I believe I am beautiful," "I will develop a healthy relationship with my body," "I will commit to my meal plan," and so forth.)

Today, I am letting go of:______________________________

(For example, grudges, certain negative thoughts, regrets, self-imposed stress, and so forth.)

My exercise plan today:_________________________________

My fasting window:_______ (Such as 8 p.m. to noon the next day.)

My daily macros: carbs ________ fats ________ protein ________

You don't need any fancy book to journal—just a notebook if writing by hand, or a dedicated file on your laptop or iPad. For further ideas, see the Daily Recharge Journal that I also created, available on my website. It has spaces for each of these topics every day.

Consider Certain Supplements

A lot of people ask me about the value of taking nutritional supplements. My response is always to emphasize, above all, that supplements are just that—they are meant to *supplement* your diet, not to replace foods. Your nutrition should come primarily from whole, natural foods, not from pills. Fruits, vegetables, and other healthy foods contain nutrients and other substances not found in pills or capsules. You just can't get that synergistic benefit from a supplement.

That said, the average American diet leaves a lot to be desired. Studies show that our meals are lacking in a number of important nutrients, including magnesium, vitamin D, and fiber. True, many of these nutrients are difficult to obtain through diet alone, and I've struggled with this issue myself.

I have designed the Galveston Diet to be high in fiber, vitamin D, magnesium, omega-3 fatty acids, and other essential nutrients. In Chapter 7, you'll learn how to select the food sources with the most nutrition. Still, you may not obtain all you need. In that case, supplements can be a buffer, making up for what might be lacking. Although you do not need supplements to be successful on the Galveston Diet, consider taking the following three supplements—just to cover your bases.

Fiber Supplements

It can be difficult to obtain all the fiber you need for good health from food alone. Trust me, I've tried! All of us need between 25 and 30 grams of fiber daily. That is a lot, so supplementation is a great option. Another reason I recommend fiber supplementation is personal. I had an uncle who died of colon cancer at age 51. He was diagnosed with the disease in his forties, and he fought it for many years before succumbing. I also have aunts, uncles, cousins, and two brothers who died of cancer. I believe something genetic is going on and that I may have a predisposition for it—which is why I want to be in the best possible position to fight cancer, should I be diagnosed with it.

Fiber may be protective against cancer. A large body of literature suggests that eating a variety of foods containing high fiber has a protective effect against colon cancer, for example. Evidence also indicates that a high fiber diet may be protective against breast, ovary, endometrial, and gastrointestinal cancer.

There are many fiber supplements available, and I offer one on my website (see Resources on page 261 or access the link there for more information). If you're considering taking a fiber supplement, here's what to look for when choosing a product:

- Check that it contains both soluble and insoluble fiber.
- Be aware of the fiber source. Some fibers are derived from natural ingredients while others are synthetic. It is better for your health and digestion to supplement with natural fibers. When formulating our company's fiber supplement, I chose natural gluten-free fibers such as buckwheat (both soluble and insoluble), chia seeds (soluble), millet (insoluble), amaranth (insoluble), and quinoa (both soluble and insoluble). Other good natural fiber sources are pectin, a soluble fiber found in fruits and berries, and psyllium, a soluble fiber from the husk of the *Plantago* genus of plants.
- Read the labels for sugar content. Many flavored fiber supplements—including powders and gummies—can contain an appalling amount of sugar. One very popular brand of psyllium husk fiber contains 16 grams of sugar per dose—that's equivalent to 4 teaspoons! You can avoid all that extra sugar by opting for

sugar-free versions of powders (make sure they're sweetened with monk fruit or stevia, not chemical sweeteners).

A word of caution: If you're not accustomed to taking fiber supplements, start slowly. Adding a lot of fiber to your diet right away can trigger some uncomfortable side effects, like bloating, cramping, and gas. Gradually build up how much you take, perhaps starting with half the recommended dose for one to two weeks, before taking the full daily dose. It also helps to take fiber supplements with a large glass of water and to stay hydrated throughout the day.

Vitamin D

The body requires sunlight to manufacture vitamin D, but as a nation, we are deficient in this vitamin. One reason for this is that we're eating fewer dairy products, which are good sources of vitamin D. Also, more and more people are sitting inside (in offices or in front of home screens) every day and not getting outside much. If you live at a latitude where sunlight is limited for part of the year, you likely won't get the vitamin D you need during that time. Or, if you live where there are long days of daily sunshine, you may be using lots of sunscreen and staying out of the sun to avoid skin cancer. And, finally, if you have darker pigmented skin, you don't absorb as much sunlight, which means you have less sunlight to convert vitamin D to its active form.

The recommended form of vitamin D is vitamin D3, or cholecalciferol, because the body absorbs it more easily.

Omega-3 Fatty Acid Supplements

I have an ongoing love affair with omega-3 fatty acids because they offer so many powerful benefits for your body and brain; I discuss these at length in Chapter 7.

Although omega-3 fatty acids are found in foods—fish, seeds, and nuts, most prominently—it can be difficult to obtain all their health benefits from food alone. This is why I recommend supplementation.

When choosing a supplement, make sure it contains eicosapentaenoic acid (EPA) and docosahexaenoic acid (DHA). These are the most effective omega-3 fats, and they are found in fatty fish and algae.

There are no official guidelines for the intake of omega-3s, but respected health organizations generally recommend a 500 mg minimum of combined EPA and DHA per day, unless instructed otherwise by a health professional.

Hot Flash: Three Things to Do—Starting Now!

If you are in perimenopause or menopause, please pay attention. As you begin the Galveston Diet (Part II), you must do three things now for your health:

- Make sure you're doing the right type and duration of exercise for your body. This is usually a combination of resistance training and cardio. If you're not currently exercising, join a workout facility, get a trainer, or set up a home workout plan for yourself. Get moving at least three times a week for 45 minutes to 1 hour each session. Studies have shown that many of the changes—both physical and mental—that we associate with aging and menopause are at least partially the result of inactivity.
- Get mentally prepared to change your nutrition. In terms of perimenopause and menopause, be aware of which foods are high in protein, antioxidants, vitamins and minerals, and fiber; for example: veggies, fruits, fish, poultry. Add these foods to your diet, if you don't already eat them on a daily basis. Cut down on empty calories from sugar, junk food, and alcohol. Drink enough water daily, too (around 64 fluid

ounces/2 quarts each day). Water carries nutrients, hormones, and oxygen to your cells and disposes of waste products through your bloodstream and lymphatic system (a network of delicate tubes throughout the body). Water also lubricates your joints, enhances your health, and makes you more energetic, physically and mentally.

- Quit smoking. There are countless health reasons why you should stop smoking. But there are even more reasons when it comes perimenopause and menopause. For one thing, female smokers have more hot flashes as they transition through menopause, and smoking can initiate early menopause owing to its impact on reducing estrogen production. The main reason for this has to do with nicotine (from smoking *and* vaping); nicotine slashes the circulating estrogen levels and leads to early menopause.

  What's more, smoking during perimenopause and menopause increases the risk dramatically for diseases such as cancer, heart disease, stroke, and osteoporosis. If you're considering hormone replacement therapy, most doctors will not even prescribe it if you smoke because of smoking's adverse effect on hormones. So, join a smoking-cessation program or ask your physician for recommendations on how to quit.

It makes sense that when your body is in a time of remarkable change you would want to give it all the additional help you can. These three actions are a great place to start.

Set Up Your World for Success

Your environment—physical and social—can have a big impact on your long-term success and play a huge role in driving positive behaviors. Environment influences your decisions, your choices, and your attitude.

Your social environment is critical for success. For example, it is important to let your family, friends, and coworkers know what you are about to do. I don't think I could have succeeded, not only in doing my early version of diet but also in developing it, had it not been for the complete support of my family.

Studies show that we reflect the behaviors of the people around us. That means it's crucial that your social circle is supportive and inspiring. Most important, it should NOT be destructive or negative, or have a tendency to sabotage your efforts. Would you consider doing the Galveston Diet with a friend? Could you find a workout buddy? However you can, surround yourself with people who are also working on improving their health, fitness, and nutrition. A lot of women who have made the Galveston Diet their new lifestyle tell me that they benefited from the support they found on my online community. Get online and join them! See Resources on page 261.

Your physical environment is equally important. Here are some easy suggestions for setting it up to support your success:

- Stock your kitchen with all the essential foods and ingredients used in *The Galveston Diet.*
- Remove the foods that tempt you and replace them with ones that support your goals. Or, buy the tempting foods only for special occasions and preferably in small quantities.
- Get into the habit of meal prepping, using the meal plans in Chapter 8 as a guide. Prepare meals and snacks ahead of time, for example. Have fresh, healthy whole foods on hand and prepped. If necessary, buy pre-cut veggies. I include some specific meal prep tips in Chapter 8.

Establishing a positive environment is an important way for you to make progress in the program. In doing so, you will control your environment before it controls you. This makes problem behaviors *inconvenient* and healthy behaviors *convenient.*

Losing weight, keeping it off, and getting healthier are not quick fixes. Nor will a quick fix keep the weight off. These quick fixes and fad diets can sometimes make the situation worse, and possibly harm your health. Optimally, the only weight you can keep off long term is weight that has been lost slowly, following a healthy diet geared to meet your needs at these midlife stages of hormonal fluctuation. So, focus on eating healthy foods and engaging in fit-friendly activities you enjoy. Yes, you can still love pizza every now and then, and have a glass of wine. Modifying your eating habits isn't meant to be restrictive; actually, it's freedom. You make healthy changes you can live with for a happier long term.

PART II

THE ACTIONS

CHAPTER 4

Action 1: Intermittent Fasting

I didn't want to adopt the practice of intermittent fasting (IF) when I first heard about it. I was skeptical. I thought it was a fad. I didn't want to give up my morning coffee the way I like to drink it, and I wasn't ready to ditch breakfast.

But because I was at work developing the Galveston Diet, I kept an open mind and dug into the research. I watched a TED Talk by Dr. Mark Mattson, who was chief of the Laboratory of Neurosciences at the National Institute on Aging, and who has done extensive research on intermittent fasting. He has stated that intermittent fasting powerfully combats inflammation. That point alone sold me on IF. I already knew that the Galveston Diet would incorporate anti-inflammatory foods, so adding intermittent fasting to the plan made perfect sense: it was one more weapon to fight inflammation.

From experience, I know that intermittent fasting is a game changer. Let's unpack how it's done and why it will help you stay leaner, healthier, and younger for longer.

What Is Intermittent Fasting?

Intermittent fasting is an eating pattern that cycles between periods of eating and of not eating (fasting). There are a number of ways to go about it. One way is the 5:2 method, in which you fast for one full day, twice a week. After your fast days, you can enjoy regular meals on the remaining 5 days.

Another method is Eat Stop Eat, meaning that you do a 24-hour fast once or twice a week. For example, you fast from dinner one day to dinner the next day. This constitutes a full 24-hour fast. Similarly, One Meal a Day (OMAD) means that you fast most of the day, then eat one large meal. It could be breakfast, lunch, or dinner. You follow this pattern of eating every day.

Another variation is alternate-day fasting. This is a full 24 hours without eating anything or only eating a small amount, followed by 24 hours of eating as usual (say, three regular meals). You simply alternate the pattern: one day of fasting, followed by one day of regular meals.

Early time-restricted feeding (eTRF) is another method. It restricts your mealtimes to the morning and early afternoon, followed by a fast that lasts the rest of the day and evening.

The 16:8 Intermittent Fast

For the Galveston Diet, I recommend the 16:8 method of intermittent fasting. This fasting/eating pattern involves taking in all your meals within an 8-hour daily window of time. You then fast, or go without food, for the following 16 hours, and much of this occurs overnight, while you're sleeping. You can repeat this cycle as frequently as you'd like, from just once or twice a week to every day, but for the greatest benefit, follow the 16:8 pattern every day of the week.

The 16:8 pattern of intermittent fasting is simple to follow; I call it "fasting made easy." It provides measurable results with minimal disruption to your diet, and is generally considered less restrictive than the other methods. Additionally, it works with just about any lifestyle. Most of the participants on the Galveston Diet online program found that 16:8 is the easiest fasting plan to stick to, because it is closest to a normal eating schedule. It also builds a daily sustainable habit, which is critical to success in the program.

The most common way to do 16:8 is to skip your normal early morning breakfast, have your first meal around noon, and finish your dinner by 8 p.m. In this way, if you end your last meal at 8 p.m. and don't eat until noon the next day, you've fasted for a full 16 hours.

But what if you usually finish your dinnertime much earlier than 8 p.m.? Don't worry: 16:8 is very flexible. As long as you maintain your eating and fasting windows, you can set it up to work for you.

Within your feeding window, on the program you eat two healthy Galveston Diet–friendly meals and two snacks, without counting calories. The 16:8 method won't work effectively, however, if you eat lots of processed foods, including those with added sugar, junk food, or refined carbs. You can drink water, black coffee, and plain tea during the fast, because fluid intake is critical when fasting.

The evidence for the health benefits of 16:8 daily fasting has been growing over the past few years. A study in the journal *Cell Metabolism* reported that this method "resulted in weight loss, reduced abdominal fat, lower blood pressure, and healthier cholesterol readings." Incidentally, it is also one of the best treatments for brain fog. (For details on the benefits of intermittent fasting, see pages 70–75.)

The Earliest Fasts

Fasting, in general, is nothing new. Many religions practice fasting as part of their rituals. Muslims fast from dawn to dusk during the month of Ramadan, and Jews, Buddhists, and Hindus traditionally fast on designated days of the week or at times throughout the calendar year. Within Christianity, fasting practices vary. The Bible does not require a specific day or time for fasting, but it does refer to fasting as a beneficial spiritual practice. Catholics fast on Ash Wednesday and Good Friday, for example, and Mormons fast on the first Sunday of each month. Religions have long emphasized that fasting is good for the soul and expresses devotion, but its health benefits were not recognized until the early 1900s, when doctors used it to treat various disorders, including diabetes, obesity, and epilepsy.

Fasting predates organized religion, though. Our hunter-gatherer ancestors were the original intermittent fasters. After successfully hunting for meat or foraging for plants, they feasted. When the hunt failed or there were no plants to gather, they fasted. As a result, they evolved to be able to fully function without food for extended periods of time. All this means that from an ancestral perspective, our bodies are genetically geared to thrive on a fast-and-feast cycle. In other words, we're wired for intermittent fasting.

The Benefits of Intermittent Fasting

When done safely, intermittent fasting offers enormous health benefits to your cells, organs, bloodstream, hormones, bodily systems, and other parts and functions of your body. Let's look at the benefits of all types of intermittent fasting.

Blood Sugar and Insulin Control

Intermittent fasting also improves insulin sensitivity and reduces insulin levels. Lower insulin levels help the body burn fat more readily. Because it improves insulin sensitivity, intermittent fasting can help reduce insulin resistance. In addition, IF has been found to lower blood sugar by 3 to 6 percent and fasting insulin levels by 20 to 31 percent—reductions that can help protect against type 2 diabetes. Such findings are important because disordered blood sugar and insulin are big drivers of inflammation.

A large study in 2018 found that nearly half the participants with type 2 diabetes were able to stop using their diabetes medication and achieve remission after adopting the habit of intermittent fasting for

12 months. That's a quite remarkable outcome when it comes to managing and controlling type 2 diabetes. (Of course, never stop or reduce any medication without first consulting your physician.)

Cellular Renewal

Researchers believe that when you practice intermittent fasting, your cells undergo a small amount of stress, which seems to continually recharge the cellular defenses against molecular damage and builds your resistance to disease. Although the word *stress* sounds like a negative, taxing the body is beneficial in much the same way as exercising stresses your muscles and heart. As long as you allow your body time to recover, it will grow stronger. There is a lot of similarity between how your body responds to the stress of physical activity and how cells respond to intermittent fasting.

One of these responses is autophagy, a rejuvenation process that goes on at the cellular level. Think of autophagy as a kind of garbage disposal system in which cells eliminate damaged molecules, including those that have been associated with Alzheimer's, Parkinson's, and other neurological diseases.

Autophagy may help many aspects of the human body, including:

- Disease prevention and reversal of age-related illnesses
- Extended longevity and anti-aging
- Immune system support

Intermittent fasting also ramps up levels of "chaperone proteins" in the cells. For perspective on this, think of proteins as the workhorses of the cells, each with its own specific task.

The primary structure for proteins inside the cells is a chain of amino acids. These proteins are only useful to the cells when their chains fold into a particular shape. Improperly folded proteins can't do their jobs; they stick together, develop clumps, and congest the cell.

Many proteins cannot fold themselves unless they get help from the chaperone proteins. Without these chaperones, the proteins can't take on their correct form and the cell's health can be compromised. But when proteins are properly folded, it's the chaperones that are calling the shots.

Chaperone proteins are also natural, free-radical scavengers inside the cells. They find disease-causing free radicals and eliminate them, thus combating cell degeneration.

Anti-Inflammation

Chronic inflammation, which underlies many diseases such as diabetes, joint problems, multiple sclerosis, and inflammatory bowel syndrome (IBS), can be reduced with intermittent fasting. One of the reasons for this has to do with the monocyte, a type of white blood cell that helps fight bacteria, viruses, and other infections in the body. In a 2019 report in the journal *Cell,* scientists reported that monocytes in the blood were less inflammatory when people and mice fasted intermittently.

Galectin-3, another substance found in the blood, is also linked to chronic inflammation. Scientists from the Intermountain Healthcare Heart Institute found that intermittent fasting can increase the levels of this protein, thereby reducing inflammation in the body.

We also know from other studies that intermittent fasting helps ease inflammatory illnesses. Many joint issues, including rheumatoid arthritis, are tied to inflammation. Drops in inflammation have been seen in patients who practice intermittent fasting, and reduced inflammation can relieve pain and help protect joints.

One of the earliest pieces of evidence showing the link between fasting and inflammation involved overweight adults with moderate asthma. They went on an alternate-day fasting program and lost 8 percent of their weight over 8 weeks. Plus, they saw a reduction in markers of inflammation and improvements in their asthma symptoms.

The anti-inflammatory benefits of IF have been found to help keep arteries clear of buildup. A 2009 study reported in the *American Journal of Clinical Nutrition* discovered that intermittent fasting (alternate-day fasting) reduced total cholesterol, the "bad" LDL cholesterol, and blood triglycerides—all risk factors for heart disease and narrowed arteries.

Brain Health

Various studies, including a 2020 report in *Brain and Behavior,* show that IF can stimulate the growth of new brain cells and signaling pathways in the brain, a process called neuroplasticity, especially in the hippocampus (the center for learning and memory).

The fact that intermittent fasting triggers the formation and release of ketones is important, too, since their release into the bloodstream has been shown to protect memory and learning, as well as slow the process of disease in the brain.

The autophagy that comes with IF clears out dying or damaged cells and toxic proteins from the brain, helping to prevent dementia.

Finally, animal studies show that brain-derived neurotrophic factor (BDNF) also increases with intermittent fasting. BDNF is important for cognitive function and mood.

Protection Against Cancer

Among women, the five most common cancers are breast, colorectal, lung, cervix, and stomach cancers. Of these, breast cancer is considered the second most common cancer in the world.

A review published in the *Journal of Mid-Life Health* covered reasons why intermittent fasting might offer protection against many of these cancers, primarily because it interferes with mechanisms that promote cancer and its spread. Fasting, for example, reduces inflammation, which is associated with the development and progression of cancer. Fasting also inhibits tumor growth by interfering with angiogenesis, which is the creation of new blood vessels that feed tumors. Tumors can't grow without having a blood supply; thus, fasting can potentially slow tumor growth. Fasting also fights obesity, which is a risk factor for cancer.

In addition, intermittent fasting reduces levels of a hormone called insulin-like growth factor 1 (IGF-1). Essential for normal growth and cellular activity, and produced in the liver, this hormone is naturally very important when we're young. But elevated IGF-1 seems to be associated with aging and the development of cancer as we get older. Having high levels of IGF-1 in the body is like driving a car hard and fast, with no repair or maintenance, which likely produces defects in the car's engine. In the body, IGF-1 produces defects in the cells. The result is a higher risk of cancer and age-related diseases. However, human and animal studies have consistently shown reductions in IGF-1 levels when organisms fast. It is thought that fasting makes our bodies turn off growth and concentrate more on repair and maintenance activities—and quite possibly cut the risk of certain cancers.

Gene Expression and Anti-Aging

A gene is a tiny piece of hereditary material written in code and contained within a long molecule called deoxyribonucleic acid (DNA). The genes are responsible for a lot that goes on in your body, from metabolism to immunity to longevity. When genes are "expressed," this means they are used as blueprints for making proteins that tell a cell what to do. Gene expression is thus the process by which the information contained within a gene becomes a useful product—such as a protein—that performs a specific function.

Gene expression can be stimulated (upregulated) or suppressed (downregulated) based on a number of factors. One of these factors is intermittent fasting. A 2020 study suggested that just 30 days of moderate intermittent fasting (similar to the 16:8 pattern) can lead to measurable changes in the genes that may promote human health and longevity.

Intermittent fasting has also been found to slow the degradation of DNA, which is what occurs when we age, and to accelerate DNA repair, thus slowing down the aging process.

Fasting also increases the levels of antioxidants that can help prevent the body's cells from being harmed by free radicals, which are molecules that inflict cellular damage.

Weight Control

Studies show that people who do intermittent fasting lose weight and have a lower body mass index. They are also able to maintain their weight loss.

A 2014 review study published in *Translational Research* found that this eating pattern can promote a 3 to 8 percent reduction in weight over 3 to 24 weeks, which is a significant amount compared to most weight-loss studies. The dieters also shed 4 to 7 percent of their waist circumference. This is a substantial loss of visceral fat—the dangerous kind that accumulates around your organs and can lead to disease.

All this occurs because after fasting for 12 hours or longer, you start burning stored fat for energy instead of glucose. Fatty acids are converted to ketone bodies in the liver, which are then released into the bloodstream and used by the body and brain for energy.

Importantly, intermittent fasting spares lean muscle. This is a huge plus for women in midlife, because a primary symptom associated with menopause—and aging in general—is the loss of muscle. This loss contributes to lower strength, a slower metabolism, and accelerated aging.

Intermittent fasting also alters the hormone levels to make stored body fat more accessible to burn. For example, the levels of growth hormone (GH) skyrocket when you fast intermittently, increasing as much as fivefold. The GH helps the body burn fat and create lean muscle.

The Joy of Change

Intermittent fasting was a game-changer for Kelly. At age 42, she started experiencing almost every symptom imaginable in perimenopause. She wasn't technically overweight, but she was tired, depressed, bloated, constantly hungry, and generally unhappy with her body—even though she was active and worked out.

Kelly was intrigued by intermittent fasting and what she had learned about it. She started practicing it by easing into the habit.

After a few weeks, she was consistently fasting for 16 to 18 hours a day.

Kelly reported the following: "I feel so much better. I have this energy that had been missing for a long time. I'm not hungry all the time anymore. My clothes fit better, and the bloat is gone. I feel so light and confident now."

How to Start Intermittent Fasting—and Be Successful

The first step is to learn how to do intermittent fasting properly. If you jump in too quickly, or go about it in the wrong way, you may not get the results you want. Here's how to be successful.

Begin Gradually

If you've never done IF, start gradually. When I began intermittent fasting, I began by pushing my eating window by 30 minutes. That is, I used to eat breakfast at 6:30 a.m., so I began at 7 a.m. and did that until it felt natural. I repeated that process every few days in 30-minute increments until I reached my goal of eating at noon. It took about a month, but by moving slowly, I got into the rhythm of intermittent fasting without feeling significant hunger or experiencing irritability.

Choose Your Window

After easing toward intermittent fasting, select an 8-hour window and limit your food intake to that time span. Popular time windows include:

Noon to 8 p.m. = Your eating window
8 p.m. to noon the next day = Your fasting window
10 a.m. to 6 p.m. = Your eating window

6 p.m. to 10 a.m. the next day = Your fasting window
9 a.m. to 5 p.m. = Your eating window
5 p.m. to 9 a.m. the next day = Your fasting window

Experiment to find the best times for you.

Stay Flexible

Many people choose the 16:8 pattern, but that may not work for everyone. If you find that a 14:10 or even an 18:6 works better for you, that is completely okay. The only eating pattern that works is the one that works for you and your schedule.

Consult the Meal Plans

It's important to follow the nutritional guidance offered in Chapter 7. This includes the recommended amount of protein per day. During the fat-burning period of a fast, you can be at risk of breaking down protein to use as an energy source if you're not eating enough during your eating window. Focus on eating an ample supply of protein to prevent any kind of muscle loss or breakdown during your fast.

Your body also needs a good balance of other nutrients, including fruits and vegetables and healthy, complex carbohydrate sources in the right ratios.

The Galveston Diet's meal plans and nutritional principles will help you fill up on nutrient-rich foods; they are the perfect complement to intermittent fasting. Follow these guidelines, and you'll be successful.

Stay Hydrated

Drinking plenty of water throughout the day is important, but it is extremely important during your fasting window. When you don't eat, you're missing out on the water that would be in your foods, so you'll need to drink more fluids to compensate. In addition, drinking more fluids helps keep you full during periods of fasting, as well as reducing food cravings.

Avoid Temptation

Having tempting foods around—foods that trigger your desire to overeat—will make fasting unnecessarily hard. The look and smell of foods can set off your appetite and make you crave them. It's best to remove these foods from your kitchen and other places.

Make Use of Your Spare Time

When you fast, you gain more spare time in your schedule from those times during which you'd normally be preparing food and eating it. This newfound time is the perfect opportunity to do something you love, such as reading, listening to music, or going for a walk.

Get Plenty of Sleep

Numerous studies have shown that getting a good night's sleep suppresses your appetite and tames out-of-control hunger and cravings. Shoot for 6 to 8 hours of sleep each night. Remember, the hours you sleep count toward your fasting hours, so take advantage of this no-temptation, no-hunger time!

Exercise

Exercise can increase the benefits of intermittent fasting. Light exercise enhances circulation, improves energy levels, and lifts your mood. The timing of your exercise is up to you; experiment with what times of the day work best for you and fit your schedule.

Rest and Relaxation

Make and take time for relaxation every day. It invigorates your body and mind, promotes a positive outlook, and improves your thinking and memory. In addition, a more relaxed life supports good health, which in turn leads to greater productivity and happiness.

Reward Yourself

After you hit your IF goals for the day, week, or month, reward yourself. Whether it is carving out consistent time to do something that you love, or taking a soothing bubble bath, going for a walk, calling a friend, meditating or journaling, or even getting a manicure or facial, find something that brings you joy. Rewarding yourself after reaching a goal is important! Do not discount it.

Hot Flash: 5 Big Myths About Intermittent Fasting

As with any popular trend, there are a lot of untruths floating around about intermittent fasting. To sort fact from fiction, let's debunk some of the most prevalent myths about IF.

Myth #1: Intermittent fasting just means that you skip breakfast. It's true that most people choose a window of fasting that means skipping breakfast at their usual time. However, you can schedule your eating window so you have an earlier dinner and therefore can have breakfast, even if it's just a little later in the morning. For example, if you finish eating at 6 p.m., you can break your fast and enjoy breakfast at 10 a.m. the next day. This still keeps you on the 16:8 fasting schedule. For many people, this allows greater flexibility and may align better with their hunger patterns.

Myth #2: Intermittent fasting is appropriate for anyone.

Despite its many benefits, intermittent fasting is not right for everyone. I do not advise this strategy for those with eating disorders, anyone who is currently underweight, or someone who has type 1 diabetes. In addition, you should not begin an intermittent fasting routine while you are pregnant or breastfeeding. Children and teens generally should not fast, because they are still growing. Nor is it a good idea for people newly diagnosed with diabetes, a chronic disease, in a weakened state from surgery, or while being treated for a health concern.

Myth #3: You can eat anything you want during your eating window.

Your eating window is not a time to feast on less nutritious or processed foods. It's a time to concentrate on healthy choices. Intermittent fasting is a key part of the Galveston Diet, but remember that it works synergistically with the other two actions, including healthy food choices, to give you the best results.

Myth #4: Intermittent fasting slows your metabolism.

On the contrary, fasting, especially intermittent fasting, has been shown to boost metabolism. Your metabolism is the process by which food is turned into fuel in your body. When you fast, your body is given hormonal advantages that enhance your metabolic health.

In fact, certain hormones involved in metabolism, such as norepinephrine and growth hormone, become elevated through fasting. Not only does fasting help keep the metabolically important hormones high, but it also makes you more "metabolically flexible." This means that your body can adapt to quickly burning the fuel source, such as carbohydrates or fats, that is most readily available.

Myth #5: Intermittent fasting makes you hungry.

One reason many people are resistant to intermittent fasting is that they're afraid they'll get too hungry and not be able to stick to a healthy, nutritious eating plan. It's true that when you first start intermittent fasting you might feel hungry; this is why I advise easing into it. When you gradually increase your fasting window, you'll likely find that hunger is very manageable and not something that distracts you.

Understand, too, that your two main hunger hormones, ghrelin and leptin, respond positively to intermittent fasting. Ghrelin is a key hunger hormone that signals your body to eat. Some studies suggest that intermittent fasting can decrease ghrelin, which would then make you less hungry. There's also research that says there's an increase in leptin, which is the satiety hormone; that's the hormone that says, "Hey, I'm full."

So, once you get into the full swing of intermittent fasting, you won't have to worry about hunger or cravings.

Are You Ready?

Although intermittent fasting is easy, flexible, and effective, making the commitment might feel challenging at first. You have to be open to making such a change in your life, believe in your own power to be successful, and trust that you can and will learn to incorporate it into your lifestyle.

So—are you ready to begin your fat loss and health transformation? Are you ready to feel better, think more clearly, and feel physically stronger? Are you ready to prevent disease or reverse health conditions that have crept up on you in midlife? Are you ready to create a lean, long-lived body?

If you answered yes to even one of those changes, you are indeed ready to start IF.

CHAPTER 5

Action 2: Anti-Inflammatory Nutrition

As a physician, I've had many patients who were initially unaware that something really bad was raging in their bodies: chronic inflammation. This condition can significantly increase the risk of developing diseases like arthritis, asthma, cardiovascular disease, stroke, and more. We also know that if you are overweight or obese, your body is chronically inflamed.

Here's the really great news: many recent studies have shown the power of anti-inflammatory foods to fight inflammation, control weight, and improve health. The key is simply to concentrate on anti-inflammatory nutrition. Stay the course, and the results of eating in this manner will kick in, and you'll begin to feel much better and start losing weight.

Inflammation: Acute versus Chronic

Inflammation is a normal, defensive process that allows the immune system to fight what science calls a "stimulus." That stimulus can be an injury, an infection, a foreign body, an ingested irritant, or even cancer. As a very simple example, think of a sprained ankle that gets red and swollen, or a cut on your finger that becomes tender. The redness, pain, or swelling are normal *acute* responses of the inflammatory system.

With acute inflammation, the walls of tiny capillaries widen and become more permeable, allowing white blood cells to flood the damaged tissue. As the blood flows in, the affected area swells. This places pressure on surrounding nerves and triggers pain. But once the offending stimulus has been removed or destroyed, the tissue heals.

Acute inflammation is a necessary process—one of the primary mechanisms that protect our bodies against the thousand environmental attacks we receive every day. It serves a vital role in our maintenance and repair system. Without it, we can't survive.

Chronic inflammation is something altogether different. It is a slow, ongoing, and destructive process by which the body produces chemicals that inflame tissues.

Chronic inflammation often occurs below the pain threshold, meaning the brain does not register that it is happening. It can therefore go unnoticed and unchecked by the body for very long periods of time. This is why persistent inflammation is so dangerous and plays a role in at least seven of the top ten causes of death for adults in the United States.

Take heart disease, for example, which is the leading killer of American women. Low-density lipoproteins (LDLs)—those particles of "bad" cholesterol—can travel into the inner walls of arteries. There, they provoke an inflammatory response that can create blood clots and eventually plaques that block arteries.

Another chronic condition that has been linked to inflammation is type 2 diabetes, in which people can't adequately use insulin. Over time, without treatment, their organs begin to fail as the glucose builds to dangerous levels in the blood. Researchers have found macrophages (a type of white blood cell) in the pancreas of people with type 2 diabetes. The macrophages release inflammatory molecules that impair insulin activity.

Inflammation is a possible driver in Alzheimer's disease, too. This disease results mostly from the buildup of amyloid and tau proteins in the brain. Specialized cells called microglia patrol the brain, looking for signs of infection or inflammation caused by these offending proteins. When they're found, the microglia get rid of them. In doing so, they also dispatch pro-inflammatory chemicals called cytokines that activate other microglia. Normally, this cytokine release is short-lived; but in Alzheimer's, the microglia become overactive, increasing their production of cytokines, simultaneously clearing less, and leading to brain inflammation. The result is more and more damage to brain cells, which can gradually lead to Alzheimer's disease.

For women, the decline in estrogen during perimenopause and menopause instigates inflammation in many different organs, especially the gut lining. An unhealthy gut lining may develop small cracks or holes, allowing partially digested food, toxins, and other substances to penetrate the tissues beneath it. This triggers inflammation that can lead to problems in the digestive tract and beyond—even in the bones.

The body views inflammation as a stressor, so the way it responds to the stress is to halt normal bone turnover in favor of bone loss, possibly leading to osteoporosis. In other words, *anything* that causes inflammation may have an effect on bone health.

Decreasing estrogen levels lead to other inflammatory problems, too. These include brain inflammation and a resulting cognitive decline—specifically, verbal memory (hello, brain fog). They also lead to inflammation in the muscles, which ultimately results in loss of muscle mass and strength, otherwise known as sarcopenia.

What's more, researchers believe that declining levels of estrogen cause joint pain during menopause. When you're younger, estrogen protects your joints by keeping inflammation down. As estrogen levels begin to drop off during perimenopause, however, there is less of the hormone to protect the joints, and pain is often the result.

Weight gain brought on by hormonal changes also contributes to inflammation. There is clear evidence that fat cells, especially visceral fat cells ("belly fat") around the middle of the body, add to chronic inflammation by creating extra cytokines and elevating C-reactive protein (a marker of inflammation in the blood).

Clearly, chronic inflammation is a menace, which is why understanding and controlling it has become a central focus of modern medical preventative treatment.

The Joy of Change

Every medical condition has a story, and Anna's began with some serious issues. By the time she entered midlife and turned 50, she was suffering from osteoarthritis, stenosis (a narrowing of the spine), and degenerative disc disease. She was slowly gaining weight and dealing with other symptoms. For example, her brain seemed enveloped in a gray fog, and she began getting headaches and feeling exhausted. It all added up to a weird sense that her mind and body weren't in sync.

Frustrated, worried, and confused, Anna consulted a gastrointestinal doctor and was tested for food allergies. It turned out that she had a strong sensitivity to gluten, grains, legumes, some starches, and certain additives in foods.

As I heard Anna's story, I suspected that she had a lot of inflammation going on in her body, and it was related to her diet. Fortunately, Anna realized this too, and she got onto the road to recovery by following the Galveston Diet and eliminating inflammation-causing substances from her diet.

As she told us, "My official start date was June 1, 2020, and I weighed 159.9 pounds. Today is August 20, 2020, and I am at 146.1 pounds and feeling stronger and less inflamed."

The Power of Anti-Inflammatory Nutrition

The typical American diet, in particular, features an endless rotation of processed, highly inflammatory foods. This type of eating not only fuels chronic inflammation but also damages the heart, kidneys, brain, waistline, and more.

Small wonder, then, that the most effective way to prevent and reverse the chronic inflammation associated with these diseases and aging is through good nutrition. To suppress chronic inflammation, you'll want to eat less of certain substances—or avoid them altogether.

Omega-6 Fats Versus Omega-3 Fats

I tell my patients all that time that it is essential to lower the omega-6: omega-3 ratio. But why? What is the difference between these two types of fatty acids?

Biochemically speaking, omega-3 and omega-6 are both polyunsaturated fatty acids (PUFAs). The main difference between them has to do with their chemical makeup. Omega-3 refers to the position of the final double bond in the chemical structure, which is three carbon atoms from the "omega," or tail end of the molecular chain. In omega-6 fats, the last double bond is six carbons from the tail end. From a practical standpoint, an unbalanced ratio of these fats can provoke inflammatory processes in the body.

In Paleolithic times, early humans probably evolved and thrived on a 1:1 ratio of omega-6 to omega-3 fatty acids, although we don't know for sure. However, our genes have not changed much since then. Fast-forward to modern times, and the ratio in the Western diet, on average, is an astounding 20:1. In other words, we're eating a lot more omega-6 fats in proportion to the omega-3 fats we eat.

Where are we getting so many omega-6 fats? Mostly from many refined vegetable oils, such as sunflower, corn, soybean, and cottonseed oils. They are also plentiful in many snack foods, cookies, crackers, salad dressings, and fast foods. When omega-6 fats are broken down during normal body processes, the by-products trigger inflammation in the body. The more omega-6 fats you consume, the higher your risk is for chronic inflammation—and the diseases it causes.

As harmful as too many omega-6 fats can be, they become even worse when converted from liquid to solid or semi-solid—that is, hydrogenated or partially hydrogenated—as in the production of margarine or shortening. During the hardening, they change into trans fats, which make the membranes of cells rigid, inflexible, and essentially dysfunctional. Indeed, trans fats do a lot of damage in the body. They increase inflammation, especially in people who are very overweight or obese. They depress the immune system, lower HDL cholesterol (the good kind), and raise LDL cholesterol (the dangerous kind), as well as other bad deeds.

To protect yourself against inflammation, especially from domination by omega-6 fats and trans fats, eat more foods that are rich in omega-3 fatty acids. That will counter the effects of too many omega-6 fats in your body.

You can obtain omega-3s from fatty fish, such as salmon, mackerel, and sardines, as well as some plant foods like flax seeds and walnuts. Grass-fed animals are good sources of omega-3 fatty acids, too. If you don't like fish or don't eat it very often, you might need to supplement with an omega-3 source like fish oil.

Another action to restore the intake balance between the two fats is to ease off processed seed and vegetable oils that are high in omega-6s, as well as the processed foods that contain them. Also, avoid trans fats such as margarine and shortening.

Added Sugar

By "added sugar" I mean the kind that is added during the cooking or processing of foods (such as sucrose, dextrose, or high-fructose corn syrup), products packaged as sweeteners (such as table sugar), sugars from syrups and honey, sugars from concentrated fruit juices, and the sugar you put in your own food. Added sugars do not include the naturally occurring sugars found in fruits, vegetables, and dairy foods.

In 2015, the World Health Organization recommended that no more than 10 percent—and ideally less than 5 percent—of an adult's daily calories should come from added sugar. Put into perspective, that means an average adult who eats 2,000 calories daily should consume no more than 6 teaspoons (2 tablespoons) of sugar a day, or about 25 grams—that's the amount you'd get in a generous schmear of hazelnut spread, but quite a bit less than what is in a can of non-diet cola.

But we're eating a lot more sugar. Today, the average American ingests more than 19 teaspoons ($6^1/_3$ tablespoons), or almost 80 grams, of added sugar every day!

Too much added sugar causes inflammation in multiple ways. First, after you have eaten sugar, your blood glucose spikes. When this happens, pro-inflammatory chemicals get dispersed throughout your body, fueling inflammation. Then, your body produces insulin, which itself is a pro-inflammatory hormone.

Consumed sugar also interferes with a process called phagocytosis. This occurs when white blood cells attempt to destroy foreign particles or pathogens, such as bacteria or an infected cell, by engulfing them. In humans, phagocytosis protects the body and is a vital aspect of the immune system.

The Food and Drug Administration now requires "added sugars" to be listed on the labels of all food packaging, listed under carbohydrates. This has made it a little easier to identify the added sugar in ingredient lists. But there are upwards of fifty names for sugar appearing on these labels. So, don't just look for the word *sugar.* Look for any type of sugar, syrup, nectar, or anything ending in -ose. If you avoid foods containing added sugar, especially processed foods, you'll greatly reduce your overall intake of sugar.

Hot Flash: What No One Tells You About Artificial Sweeteners

Artificial sweeteners—the kind that you add to your coffee and that manufacturers add to packaged foods—can trigger inflammation by promoting pro-inflammatory changes in gut bacteria. Basically, artificial sweeteners cause previously healthy gut bacteria to become diseased. Then they invade the gut wall and make it more porous and leaky—a situation that potentially leads to serious health issues.

Read food labels carefully, because artificial sweeteners are lurking in many foods. You probably know the brand names of typical artificial sweeteners, but manufacturers often list them under their generic names on food labels. Aspartame, sucralose, and acesulfame-K (ace-K) are examples of generic names you may find listed.

But here's another thing that may not be common knowledge: as you taper off your use of artificial sweeteners, your taste buds get a chance to relearn what real sweetness is, and they'll thank you for it! Eventually, you'll start to enjoy the natural sweetness of real foods rather than the overpowering sweetness of processed food products and diet drinks.

Added Nitrites and Nitrates in Processed Foods

Nitrites and nitrates are both forms of nitrogen. The difference between them lies in their chemical structures: nitrates have three oxygen atoms, while nitrites have two oxygen atoms. Both nitrates and nitrites occur naturally in certain vegetables, like leafy greens, celery, and cabbage.

Although the nitrites and nitrates that occur naturally in vegetables can be helpful, there are also synthetic versions of both compounds, and these are added to foods such as cured meats (bacon, ham, hot dogs, deli meats) as preservatives. After you ingest these chemicals, they can form compounds called nitrosamines, which are inflammation-generating chemicals that can cause many types of cancer. Man-made nitrites and nitrates are harmful to the body and should be avoided.

One other big problem with these processed foods is that they trigger the formation of advanced glycation end products (AGEs), which, you guessed it, increase inflammation in the body. So, it's best to cut back on processed meats and eat them only sparingly, if at all. You can also purchase nitrate-free, uncured meats.

Artificial Colors, Flavorings, and Preservatives

If you read the ingredient label of just about any food in your kitchen pantry, in your fridge, or at the supermarket, you'll spot lots of food additives. Thousands and thousands of additives are put into various foods and food products. They're used to enhance the flavor, appearance, or texture of a product, or to extend its shelf life.

The problem with additives is that the body does not recognize them as food. Instead, they are viewed as foreign. Your body then creates inflammation as part of an immune response to defend against what it perceives as an invader.

The simplest ways to avoid food additives is to reduce your intake of processed foods, make more foods from scratch, and buy organic foods as much as possible.

Fried Foods

You might love fried foods, but your body doesn't! The oil used to fry foods is usually high in omega-6 fatty acids. Eating fried foods on a regular basis can then upset the ratio between omega-3 and omega-6 fats, which—as we have discussed—triggers inflammation.

In addition, many fried foods—like French fries and potato chips—are deep-fried at extremely high temperatures, a process that gives off an inflammatory chemical called acrylamide. The National Toxicology

Program's Report on Carcinogens considers acrylamide to be a possible carcinogen.

I admit that nothing beats the mouthwatering crunch of hot fried foods. But there are alternatives that allow us to keep the crunch but lose the bad fats and toxins in fried foods: oven-bake your fries and other dishes, or try air-frying (one study showed that air-frying lowers the amount of acrylamide in fried potatoes by 90 percent).

Saturated Fats

When I was a geologist working for an oil company, I used to go out to lunch with my coworkers. This was more than 25 years ago, when the keto and ultra-low-carb diets hit the scene and were all the rage. A few of my work buddies were on these diets, so at lunch I'd watch them eat hamburgers (no buns) piled with bacon and cheese or they would wolf down big slabs of steak but never any vegetables. They were losing weight, for sure, but at what cost with all that saturated fat?

Cheese, fatty beef, and butter all contain a lot of saturated fat, which is highly inflammatory when eaten in excess. That inflammation occurs in a couple of different ways. First, saturated fat can stimulate inflammation through molecules called toll-like receptors (TLR). Under normal circumstances, TLRs form an elite force that screens potential invaders in the body to see if they're bacterial, viral, or fungal. If they find evidence of any of these invaders, they signal the immune system to mount an attack. One of the TLR weapons, TLR4, is designed to sense bacteria.

Unfortunately, this protective mechanism can go wrong if TLR4 is exposed to too much saturated fat. When this happens, TLR4 sends the wrong signal, recognizing saturated fat as the invader. This sets off inflammation, particularly in the gut, that breaks down the gut lining, leading to leaky gut. In that situation, harmful substances escape from the gut, contributing to immune problems and poor infection control.

Saturated fat also stimulates the production of inflammatory agents called prostaglandins and leukotrienes. These can cause widespread destruction of joints and the inflammation associated with artery clogging. A high intake of saturated fats is associated with obesity, which also feeds the inflammatory process.

Additionally, women need to be aware that if they eat a lot of saturated fat, it influences their hormones, which may promote breast cancer. Excess saturated fat can generate higher levels of circulating estradiol, a potential cancer promoter when abnormally elevated in the body.

You don't have to entirely eliminate saturated fats on the Galveston Diet. As you will see in the pages ahead, I suggest you exercise a little caution and balance your intake of saturated fats with healthy fats such as olive oil, coconut oil, avocados, and so forth.

There are number of easy nutritional hacks to help you reduce and manage your intake of saturated fats:

- Eat leaner cuts of beef and pork, and trim as much visible fat as possible.
- Enjoy more fish and chicken.
- Choose a 90/10 blend for ground beef, or consider substituting ground turkey or chicken for ground beef.
- Remove the skin from chicken before cooking.
- Instead of sour cream, try a full-fat plain yogurt or a whip of yogurt and a full-fat cottage cheese.
- In recipes, use cheeses that are naturally lower in saturated fat, such as cottage cheese, ricotta cheese, Parmesan, feta, or goat cheese.

Remember to always check those food labels on reduced-fat products to be sure any fat removed has not been replaced with sugar or other unsavory ingredients!

Excessive Alcohol

Chronic heavy drinking—more than five to seven drinks weekly—tends to disrupt the balance between the "good" and "bad" bacteria in your gut. This imbalance creates inflammation and steals the health of your immune system. Alcohol also promotes the overgrowth of bad bacteria, which further harms your gut, weakening its lining. The gut then becomes porous and allows harmful bacteria and toxins to leak out into the bloodstream to reach the organs. Excessive alcohol use on a regular basis can also lead to organ damage.

It's wise to restrict your alcohol consumption to about one drink a day. This translates to one 5-ounce glass of wine, a 12-ounce bottle of beer, or 1.5 ounces of hard liquor.

Is Your Body Inflamed?

Take this quiz to determine your relative degree of inflammation based on your nutritional choices for one day, or the past 24 hours. You can take this quiz as many times as you'd like. The goal is to get as low a score as possible. This then indicates your nutritional choices are decreasing your body's chronic inflammation rather than promoting it.

How much alcohol did you consume during this time?

a. None
b. One drink
c. More than one drink

How many servings of whole fruit did you have?

1 serving = 1 apple, 1 cup berries, etc.

a. More than 1 serving
b. 1 serving
c. None

How many servings of leafy veggies did you have?

1 serving = 1 cup raw

a. More than 1 serving

b. 1 serving

c. None

How many servings of beans or legumes did you have?

1 serving = 1/2 cup cooked

a. More than 1 serving

b. 1 serving

c. None

How many servings of seafood did you have?

1 serving = 6 ounces cooked

a. More than 1 serving

b. Serving

c. None

How many servings of other veggies (tomatoes, carrots, peas, zucchini, squash, etc.) did you have?

1 serving = 1 cup raw

a. More than 1 serving

b. 1 serving

c. None

How many servings of nuts and seeds did you have?

1 serving = 1/4 cup

a. More than 1 serving

b. 1 serving

c. None

How much fiber did you consume?

a. 25–35 grams

b. 20–25 grams

c. Less than 20 grams

How much omega-3 fats did you have?

1 serving = 6 ounces fatty fish (salmon, mackerel, tuna, etc.), cooked; or omega-3 supplement

a. More than 1 serving

b. 1 serving

c. None

How much green or black tea did you have?

1 serving = 1 cup

a. More than 1 serving

b. 1 serving

c. None

How much olive oil did you consume?

a. 2–3 tablespoons

b. 1 tablespoon

c. None

Eating the rainbow! Count the number of different colors you have consumed from fruits and veggies throughout the day.

a. 2 colors or more

b. 1 color

c. None

Did you use any garlic, ginger, fresh herbs, or turmeric?

Fresh only

a. More than 1 use

b. 1 use

c. None

Did you have an avocado? How much?

a. Whole

b. ½

c. None

Did you consume any fermented products (yogurt, kombucha, etc.)?

a. 2 servings

b. 1 serving

c. None

How much added sugar (in grams) did you consume?

Read food labels and total the gram amounts

a. Less than 25 grams

b. 25–50 grams

c. More than 50 grams

How many sugar-sweetened beverages did you consume?

1 serving = 12 ounces

(including soda, sweet tea, juices, etc.)

a. None

b. 1 serving

c. More than 1 serving

How many servings of refined grains did you consume?

1 serving = 1 slice white bread, ½ cup cooked white rice or noodles, etc.

a. None or 1 serving

b. 2 servings

c. 3 or more servings

How many servings of red meat did you consume?

1 serving = 3 ounces cooked, lean

a. None

b. 3 ounces or less

c. 4 ounces or more

How much artificial sweetener did you consume?

a. None

b. 1 serving

c. More than 1 serving

How much trans fat did you consume?

(shortening, partially hydrogenated vegetable oil, margarine)

a. None

b. 1 serving

c. More than 1 serving

How much processed meat (with preservatives and nitrates) did you consume?

(luncheon meats, hot dogs, bacon)

a. None

b. 1 serving

c. More than 1 serving

How much fried food did you consume?

1 serving = 3 ounces

a. None

b. 1 serving

c. More than 1 serving

How much junk food did you consume?

(fast foods, convenience foods, potato chips, pretzels, etc.)

a. None

b. 1 serving

c. More than 1 serving

How much vegetable oil containing omega-6 fats did you consume?

(safflower oil, sunflower oil, corn oil, soybean oil, etc.)

a. 1 tablespoon

b. 2–3 tablespoons

c. 4–6 tablespoons

How much food containing artificial additives (colors, flavors, preservatives) did you consume?

1 serving = $1/2$ cup

(artificial flavors, colors, chemical preservatives, etc.)

a. None

b. 1 serving

c. More than 1 serving

Scoring

Review your answers. For each (a) you selected, give yourself 0 points. For each (b), give yourself 1 point. For each (c), give yourself 2 points. Add up your total.

Very low inflammation in your body: 0–15

Moderate inflammation in your body: 16–30

High inflammation in your body: 31–50

Focus on Foods That Heal

This chapter has covered the main foods that cause chronic inflammation. Let's now get acquainted with the foods that actively fight inflammation in the body! These are the heart and soul of the Galveston Diet.

Some of the best tools to combat chronic inflammation comes not from the pharmacy but from the grocery store. Much research has found that components of some foods or beverages have anti-inflammatory effects, and you'll enjoy most of these foods on the Galveston Diet.

Among the most powerful of these components are the antioxidants, valued for their potential in fighting cellular damage. An antioxidant is a substance that protects cells from the damage caused by free radicals. A free radical is a molecule that has lost part of itself—that is, it has lost one of its electrically charged electrons that normally orbit in pairs. To restore that balance, the radical steals an electron from nearby molecules.

In doing so, it inflicts damage on cell membranes, leaving those cells to disintegrate. Thus, the production of free radicals leads to various inflammatory-associated diseases.

But we have antioxidants to the rescue! Research shows that antioxidants may help prevent certain cancers, reduce cholesterol levels, and increase immune function. They donate an electron to a free radical without becoming harmed in the process. Antioxidants thus put an end to the destructive, pro-inflammatory rampage of free radicals.

Vitamin antioxidants include vitamins A, C, and E, while mineral antioxidants include zinc, selenium, copper, and manganese. Inflammation-fighting foods to choose for these antioxidants include the following:

- Blueberries, blackberries, raspberries, strawberries, and cranberries are on the A-list as sources of fruit-derived antioxidants.
- Artichokes, kale, and bell peppers are among the richest sources of antioxidants in veggies. Other powerful sources include asparagus, beets, broccoli, red cabbage, and tomatoes.
- Walnuts, pistachios, pecans, hazelnuts, and almonds are high in antioxidants, as are seeds.
- Legumes—such as kidney beans, edamame, and lentils—pack an antioxidant punch.
- Many spices have amazing antioxidant characteristics, especially cloves, garlic, ginger, turmeric, and any fresh herb.
- Coffee, tea, and red wine (in moderation) are rich in antioxidants.
- Foods rich in omega-3 fatty acids are powerful sources of anti-inflammatory components. These include fish such as salmon and mackerel. (If fish is not an option or you don't eat it often or at all, supplementing with fish oil is a good plan B.)

To enrich your diet with antioxidants, shoot for variety. No one single food or food group should be your sole priority. Instead, incorporate lots of different fruits, vegetables, nuts, legumes, and spices into your diet.

The Galveston Diet meal plans (see Chapter 8) will lend a healthy variety to your eating. They will provide you with a framework for your meals and will inspire you to create your own meals and snacks.

Hot Flash: My Favorite Anti-Inflammatory Foods

Asparagus
Avocados
Beans and other legumes
Beets
Berries
Broccoli
Carrots
Celery
Kale
Olive oil
Oranges
Pineapple
Salmon
Shiitake mushrooms
Spinach
Sweet potatoes
Swiss chard
Tomatoes
Walnuts

Whether you're aiming to ease perimenopause and menopause symptoms, lose weight, or prevent cancer, heart disease, diabetes, dementia, or other conditions connected to chronic inflammation, *the sooner you shift to anti-inflammatory nutrition, the better*!

CHAPTER 6

Action 3: Fuel Refocus

I've met many women who were literally addicted to processed carbohydrates, especially foods high in added sugar. They'd sprinkle sugar on their already sugary cereal in the morning, snack on chocolate nibs throughout the day, and eat ice cream after dinner. They just didn't seem to be able to get enough sweets.

And no wonder. Sugar is lurking everywhere, and its lure is powerful. Most food manufacturers don't make it easy on us. In fact, they are at the root of the sugar problem. There are more than 600,000 processed foods in grocery stores, 80 percent of which contain added hidden sugar. As I mentioned earlier, the average American consumes 19 teaspoons of sugar a day. One serving of a popular commercial pasta sauce has more sugar than a serving of Oreo cookies! Sweetened yogurts may be filled with more sugar than a can of soda.

Debate has raged recently about whether junk food—the super-processed, ultra-palatable stuff—is addictive in the same way that heroin or cocaine is addictive. After all, many people often feel overwhelmed with cravings that drive them to seek out sweets and devour them in a flash. Well, the verdict is starting to come in: a 2018 study found that higher sugar, higher glycemic foods can indeed be addictive—and in animal studies, they have been shown to be more addictive than cocaine.

Naturally, there are consequences—serious ones. Processed carbohydrates and added sugar are considered the main detrimental additives in our diets. They're often cited as the lead contributors to various chronic, inflammation-related illnesses, from obesity to diabetes to Alzheimer's disease.

Today, a growing body of science suggests that those who are overweight, obese, pre-diabetic or diabetic, or even addicted to processed carbs might do best on a diet that is higher in total fat and lower in carbohydrates. In fact, the proof is overwhelmingly in favor of limiting carbohydrates, increasing good fats, and eating moderate amounts of protein.

This is exactly what the Fuel Refocus phase of the Galveston Diet is all about.

What Is Fuel Refocus?

Our bodies prefer to burn glucose for fuel, derived from the carbohydrates in our diets through a process called gluconeogenesis, which takes place in the liver. Once our sources of glucose are burned up, our bodies then switch to burning body fat for fuel.

But remember, the American diet is loaded with carbohydrates (e.g., bread, pasta, rice, desserts, and added sugars). These flood the body with glucose, which stimulates insulin release. Insulin is the main hormonal driver of fat storage in the body. So, when you eat that way, your body never switches into fat *burning* mode and yet also stores more of it! It's a lose-lose situation.

To combat this, it's vital to refocus your macros (protein, carbohydrates, and fat) and adjust your percentages to those that activate fat burning and stimulate the body to rely on fat as its main source of fuel. When you refocus your macros and adjust your percentages away from the typical American diet and toward percentages that encourage fat burning, your body creates ketone bodies in the process. These fatty acids are a form of fuel that help the body burn fat, instead of using glucose (sugar) from carbs.

This biochemistry is the essence of Action 3: Fuel Refocus.

The Macros in Fuel Refocus

The macronutrient ratio of the typical American diet is as follows: 50 percent of calories from carbohydrates, 15 percent from protein, and 35 percent from fat.

We're going to change that. On the Galveston Diet, you'll adjust your macros to enhance fat burning, fueling your body with healthy fats and protein and high-quality carbs in percentages that encourage the body to utilize fat for fuel. Those percentages are as follows: 70 percent healthy fats, 20 percent lean protein, and 10 percent carbohydrates.

The daily meal plans in this program are calibrated for these macros, so it's easy to meet your macro goals. When you begin to plan meals on your own, you can track your own macros using your nutrition tracker (see page 55).

Here's an overview of the approved options to help you meet your macros.

70 Percent Healthy Fats

These include avocado, avocado oil, coconut oil, olive oil, olives, seeds (especially chia and flax seeds), butter, raw nuts (especially almonds, macadamia nuts, pecans, and walnuts), nut butters (no sugar added), and mayonnaise (olive oil or avocado oil based).

20 Percent Lean Protein

Choose from grass-fed animal protein (beef, bison, chicken, lamb, pork, turkey), wild-caught fish and seafood, anchovies, sardines, eggs, nitrate-free beef jerky, and protein powder (limited ingredient, low sugar, low-carb).

10 Percent Carbohydrates

Carbohydrates are generally classified as two types, complex and simple. Complex carbohydrates are high-fiber foods, which improve your digestion and overall gut health. They also help stabilize your blood sugar, keep your energy at an even level, and help you feel satisfied longer after meals. They are less likely to be deposited as fat.

Examples of complex carbs are vegetables, legumes, fruits, and whole grains. My favorites are apples, artichokes, asparagus, bell peppers, beets, berries, broccoli, broccoli slaw, Brussels sprouts, cauliflower, leafy greens, nuts and seeds, and pickles. These are carbs to enjoy.

Carbs to avoid are simple carbs. These are smaller molecules of sugar that are digested quickly by the body. They cause a rapid spike in insulin. If not burned off right away, they can be converted to body fat. They are typically found in foods rich in added sugars or processed white flour that has been stripped of fiber and nutrients. Examples are candy and other sweets, bread and other baked goods, and various processed foods.

Once you begin the Galveston Diet for Life program, in Chapter 10—which guides you through maintenance—you'll refocus your fuel again but over several weeks in order to stabilize your weight and increase your intake of anti-inflammatory foods. For example, you'll:

1. Start with one or more weeks at 60 percent fat, 20 percent protein, and 20 percent carbohydrates.
2. Progress to additional weeks at 50 percent fat, 20 percent protein, and 30 percent carbohydrate.
3. Stabilize long term at 40 percent fat, 20 percent protein, and 40 percent carbohydrates. These percentages are those that you'll

use forever, after you've reached a size you like and are feeling really healthy and energetic.

There's lots to look forward to!

Hot Flash: Meet Your Carbohydrate Macronutrient Goals with Low-Starch Veggies

As you track your carbohydrate macros, understand that there are two main categories of vegetables: starchy and non-starchy. Starchy veggies include sweet potatoes, corn, beans, and legumes (beans, peas, lentils), while non-starchy types include broccoli, cauliflower, tomatoes, and zucchini.

Both starchy and non-starchy vegetables are complex carbohydrates, but as the category names indicate, the key distinction between the two lies in their total starch content. Cooked starchy vegetables, such as potatoes, pack about 15 grams of carbs and 80 calories per ½ cup, whereas non-starchy types like broccoli contain about 5 grams of carbs and 25 calories in an equivalent portion. Also, starchy vegetables can raise your blood sugar levels faster than non-starchy veggies.

Although both forms of carbs are high in fiber, antioxidants, vitamins, and minerals, if weight loss is your goal, you will want to want to modify your intake of starchy vegetables in order to achieve your daily carb macros and burn fat steadily.

The table on page 106 lists some examples from both categories.

Starchy	Non-Starchy	
Corn	Artichokes	Cucumbers
Parsnips	Asparagus	Eggplant
Peas	Green beans	Mushrooms
Plantain	Italian beans	Onions
Potatoes	Peppers (all)	Broccoli
Squash	Salad greens	Brussels sprouts
Sweet potatoes	Cauliflower	Spinach
Succotash	Kale	Sprouts
Yams	Carrots	Wax beans
	Zucchini	Tomatoes

The Important Distinction Between Net Carbs and Total Carbs

On the Galveston Diet, you'll be tracking net carbs. Net carbs are the total grams of carbohydrates in any given food minus its grams of fiber.

There's a pretty simple and easy way to figure this out. If you look at the Nutrition Facts label of a given food, you'll see the total carbohydrates per serving are listed. Indented under total carbohydrates, you'll find the amount of fiber and the amount of total sugar, which includes added sugars. All these components make up the total carbohydrate number, but because fiber is not absorbed in the digestive process, we'll subtract them from the total:

Total carbohydrates - Fiber = Net carbohydrates

The idea behind using net carbs is that our body digests each type of carbohydrate differently. Net carbs are the carbohydrates that you digest and use for energy; as mentioned, the remaining fiber passes through the digestive tract without being absorbed and thus does not elevate your blood sugar. Low-net-carb foods do not have a significant impact on your blood sugar and are therefore likely to help support weight loss.

Nutrition Facts	
8 servings per container	
Serving size	**2/3 cup (55g)**
Amount per serving	
Calories	**230**
	% Daily Value*
Total Fat 8g	**10%**
Saturated Fat 1g	**5%**
Trans Fat 0g	
Cholesterol 0mg	**0%**
Sodium 160mg	**7%**
Total Carbohydrate 37g	**13%**
Dietary Fiber 4g	**14%**
Total Sugars 12g	
Includes 10g Added Sugars	**20%**
Protein 3g	
Vitamin D 2mcg	10%
Calcium 260mg	20%
Iron 8mg	45%
Potassium 235mg	6%

* The % Daily Value (DV) tells you how much a nutrient in a serving of food contributes to a daily diet. 2,000 calories a day is used for general nutrition advice.

Calculating Net Carbs

Remember, to calculate net carbs you simply subtract the grams of fiber from the grams of total carbohydrates. For the food whose nutritional label is given above, 37 grams (total carbohydrate) minus 4 grams (dietary fiber) equals 33 grams (net carbs).

The Common Challenges with Fuel Refocus

As you refocus your macros, you may be worrying that you'll miss pasta or bread or potatoes, or you'll worry about your sweet tooth getting the best of you. But let me reassure you. Your cravings will fall off (along with pounds and inches), you'll feel more energized, and healthier, and you'll feel completely satiated on the Galveston Diet. I can say this with confidence because so many women I've heard from have told me so!

Still, it's important to understand that your body has been fueled by carbohydrates for most of your life. You are now asking your metabolism to switch from burning carbs to burning stored fat—which means you're likely to face a few challenges. But don't get discouraged! You are not alone in feeling some or all the following as you get started on the Galveston Diet.

Impatience with Fat Adaptation

When you start the program you'll be training your body to adapt to burning fat as its main fuel source rather than carbohydrates. This doesn't happen overnight, however. Studies show that becoming fat-adapted happens over weeks, not days. Most people actually need three to four weeks to reach peak fat-burning adaptation. What this means as a practical matter is that you may not see or feel big results for several weeks. Be patient! Once your body adapts to burning fat, the changes will come fast!

Carbohydrate Withdrawal

If you've been eating lots of complex carbs, you can expect some changes to your mood and energy levels when you switch your macronutrient intake to 10 percent carbohydrates. Indeed, this restriction can produce some withdrawal effects in the early stages. For instance, you may experience:

- fatigue
- headaches
- cough
- sniffles
- irritability
- nausea

Ironically, if you experience any of these symptoms, it's actually a good sign. It means that at one time your body was dependent on burning glucose for fuel. Now your metabolism is shifting to rely on fat for fuel. You are simply going through withdrawal from sugar and high-carbohydrate foods and are moving into fat-burning mode (fat adaptation!).

Carbohydrate withdrawal is not fun, but hang in there. You can minimize the side effects, even if you can't eliminate them completely. One of the best ways is to replenish your electrolytes. Electrolytes include important minerals such as magnesium, potassium, sodium, calcium, phosphorus, and chloride, and they are vital in that they enable cells to generate energy, maintain the stability of their membranes, and function optimally in general. They also generate electricity, assist muscle contraction, transport water and fluids within the body, and participate in many other activities.

You can replenish your electrolytes by drinking adequate water throughout the day and introducing foods that are high in electrolytes into your diet.

To get enough potassium, for example, enjoy lots of green leafy vegetables and avocados. Honestly, I recommend eating at least one avocado a day. As for magnesium, nuts such as walnuts, almonds, pistachios, and pecans, as well as pumpkin and sunflower seeds, are wonderful sources and easy to add to any meal or snack.

Other electrolytes (especially calcium) are plentiful in green vegetables, and you can get sodium and chloride from gently salting your foods. Proteins such as tuna and chicken are rich in phosphorus.

Not Getting Enough Fat

Perhaps in the past you've been told to cut back on fats. But on this plan, fat is your new energy source. You need it. If you don't get enough fat, your energy levels will suffer, and this plan may become difficult.

The best way to think of the Galveston Diet is that it's not simply a lower-carb diet; it's a high-healthy-fat diet. You may need to change your mindset from "eliminate carbs" to "get enough fat."

With Fuel Refocus, about 70 percent of your calories should come from fat; that means enjoying foods such as eggs, uncured bacon, nuts, seeds, avocados, avocado oil, olive oil, coconut oil, and butter.

Avoiding Hidden Carbs

Carbs and added sugar are sneaky, and avoiding them can be quite a challenge. Many foods hide significantly more sugar and processed carbohydrates than you might realize, so it is important not only to read the nutrition labels but also to understand how the food was prepared and figure out how many carbs you're eating.

Carbs aren't just lurking in the obvious foods; they're also hiding out in seemingly innocent foods. Here's a short list of places where you'll find hidden carbs and added sugar:

Reduced-fat foods
Liquid eggs
Sauces
Condiments
Peanut butter
Salad dressings
Protein and energy bars

Hot Flash: Carb Swaps for Success

Here are some delicious substitutions for high-carb foods that will help you reach and maintain your carb macro goal of 10 percent.

High-Carb Food	Low-Carb Swap
Bread	Lettuce wraps or low-carb tortillas
Breading	Grated cheese or almond flour
Chips	Parmesan cheese crisps
Mashed potatoes	Mashed cauliflower
Pasta	Zoodles or other spiralized non-starchy vegetables
Rice	Cauliflower rice
Soda	Sparkling water
Wheat flour	Almond flour

Consuming Enough Protein

The challenge of eating enough protein is in figuring out when you should eat it.

Most people eat protein at just one meal—say, dinner—but to maintain muscle at any age, it's best to eat your protein throughout your 8-hour feeding window. This helps prevent muscle loss, which is important for women approaching and entering midlife. It also helps the hormones that control hunger and satiety, leptin and ghrelin, stay in balance.

And you don't have to necessarily eat protein after a workout. You may have heard that protein is needed 30 minutes to 1 hour after exercising. I believed this advice for years, until I found out that it was based on a study involving 25-year-old male athletes. Those subjects who took in protein within 30 minutes of working out gained more muscle mass when compared to those who did not (although they still gained muscle, just not as much). These findings are irrelevant to us because they apply to young men. Plus, most of us are not looking to gain a crazy amount of muscle.

For some guidelines, aim to eat 25 to 30 grams of protein, or 3 ounces, at each of your meals and 10 to 20 grams of protein, or 1.5 ounces, for your snacks. Be sure to have your protein along with healthy fats and carbs to promote fullness.

Don't overdo your protein intake, however; that is, don't exceed these recommendations. If there is excess amino acid floating around in your bloodstream, your body will convert it to glucose to use for fuel, defeating the body's ability to burn fat.

Get Off Sugar in 10 Days—My Sugar Detox

Our bodies get used to a certain amount of sugar. The more sugar we eat, the more sugar we crave, and I'm talking about "added sugar"—the type that is added during the processing of foods, as well as table sugar, honey, syrups, or any sugars that we add to our food. The good news is that it's possible to reverse that trend and eliminate your sweet tooth.

The proof for this is in a study published in the *American Journal of Clinical Nutrition.* The researchers enlisted 29 volunteers who habitually drank at least two sugar-sweetened beverages a day. As part of the experiment, the volunteers were asked to rate the sweetness of some sweetened puddings and drinks. The researchers then asked half the people to cut back on their sugar by 40 percent, and they allowed the other half to continue with their regular diets.

After three months, the people in the study went back to eating whatever they wanted to eat for a month. The researchers asked the participants to rate the sweetened puddings and beverages again. The people who had lowered their intake of sugar thought the pudding and beverages were too sweet and liked them less. They had actually lost their desire for sweets!

If you have a sweet tooth, this means that after you wean yourself off sugar, it loses its addictive grip on you. To get you started on that, try my 10-day sugar detox and repeat as necessary.

Day 1. In your journal, write down your goals for breaking your sugar addiction. For example:

- Curb my intake of added sugar.
- Educate myself on the health consequences of eating too much sugar.
- Take action each day to break my addiction, such as:
    - Focusing on whole, unprocessed foods.
    - Swapping sodas, juices, sweet tea, and other sugary drinks with water or unsweetened seltzer.
    - Drinking coffee black as a part of intermittent fasting.
    - Sweetening plain Greek yogurt with fresh or frozen berries instead of buying flavored, sugar-loaded yogurt.
    - Consuming whole fruits instead of sugar-sweetened foods or desserts.
    - Replacing candy with a homemade trail mix of fruit and nuts.

Day 2. Starting today, track your added sugar intake in your app. You may be really surprised by the total amounts you start to see. Remember, for women, the American Heart Association recommends no more than 25 grams of added sugars per day. Seeing how much more than that you are regularly consuming can be shocking—and motivating!

Day 3. If you're still drinking soft drinks, sweetened tea or coffee, sweet cocktail mixers, commercial juices, and so forth, start drinking carbonated waters infused with citrus fruit or cucumbers instead. Take the additional step of getting rid of all sweetened beverages you've got in the house.

Day 4. Stress affects your food choices and amplifies your cravings for sweets, so you'll want to do stress-relieving activities like yoga and meditation. Also, reach for high-magnesium foods, since magnesium helps calm the body. Examples are apples, avocados, or almonds. Have those with an egg or two (rich in brain-friendly vitamins) or fatty fish (packed with depression-lifting omega-3 fatty acids).

Day 5. Foods high in added sugar, such as packaged foods loaded with high-fructose corn syrup (HFCS), feed your addiction and fuel your hunger and cravings for more. Today, start creating satiating meals and snacks by pairing a healthy carb with protein or a healthy fat. Instead of a cookie or handful of crackers or chips, for example, try pairing an apple with a small handful of almonds or yellow squash plus hummus.

Day 6. Start a label-reading habit if you haven't begun already. Remember, many foods and condiments are sneaky sources of processed carbs and added sugar. Check the labels of products like salad dressings, condiments, sauces, and other foods to scan for sneaky carbs.

Day 7. Can't yet ditch your usual sugary dessert? Ask yourself: Are you actually hungry or is your nightly sugar fix a hard-to-break habit? If you're truly hungry, prepare something high in protein with a healthy fat—say, a handful of walnuts or unsweetened Greek yogurt with berries and unsweetened coconut. This kind of combo can replace your nightly dessert in a highly satisfying way.

Day 8. Little-known fact: Drinking ample water each day can help you manage sugar cravings. What's ample? Aim for 64 fluid ounces a day; that's 8 cups a day. Feel free to add some citrus or fresh herbs to your water to make it more interesting.

Day 9. Time to ease off artificial sweeteners, too. They may seem like a good idea while you're getting off the added sugar, but they can mess up your efforts. Research suggests that artificial sweeteners may promote metabolic changes that actually *increase* cravings, food intake, and weight gain. Start easing off these sweeteners by using half the amount you've been accustomed to and halve that amount again every couple of days. If you still need some sweetness, switch to stevia or erythritol.

Day 10. Congratulations—you're really on your way. You're likely already craving sweets a whole lot less, and maybe you've weaned yourself off added sugars entirely. Keep halving the amount of artificial sweeteners you've been using or ingesting. Keep drinking lots of water. And reflect on the goals you set out at the beginning of this 10-day process. Record your successes in your journal and write down how you feel, now that you've cut back on or eliminated added sugars.

The truth is that sugar isn't required in any diet. You must consume protein. You must consume quality carbs. You must consume healthy fat. You don't need to consume any sugar. The Galveston Diet was developed with these facts in mind. And the program will help you break your sugar addiction. I promise you can do it. Once you do, your love affair with added sugar will be a thing of the past.

PART III

THE PLAN

CHAPTER 7

The Galveston Diet Nutritional Foundation

The body you're feeding at age 40, 50, 60, or beyond is hardly the same body you nourished at age 20. With perimenopause and menopause, and then postmenopause, everything is changing—your shape, body composition, metabolism, muscles, bones, and energy, as well as your outer appearance and your overall health. Because of these changes, you need specific foods and nutrients not only for weight loss but also for optimal health for the long run.

Many of us don't think about turning to food first as a remedy for the issues that affect us now. More often, we look to medication for help. But fortunately, we *can* select the foods that support our hormones, fuel our bodies, and lessen, reverse, and even alleviate our symptoms.

After guiding tens of thousands of women like you through this program, I've seen direct evidence that the Galveston Diet is the surest way to better health at midlife, with fewer symptoms and permanent weight loss. You're going to be pleasantly surprised at the healing power of this diet!

What thousands of women have discovered is that eating *the right foods in the right ratios* is powerful medicine; the results will help your weight, your hormones, any chronic inflammation, and your overall health.

With this in mind, let's look at everything you get to eat—and why.

Healthy Fats

Dietary fat is not the bad guy we've been led to believe. In the late 1970s, it was popular to demonize fat. In fact, fat took the rap for causing everything from high cholesterol to diabetes, heart disease, and obesity. As a result, low-fat foods popped up everywhere! But the problem with these foods was that they lacked essential, naturally occurring nutrients and left you feeling hungry. How did this happen? Food manufacturers added—you guessed it—sugar for flavor, and so began the downfall of our health.

So, welcome back, fat. On the Galveston Diet, you'll enjoy plenty of healthy, "good" fats. These fats can reduce the risk of heart attack and stroke, support brain function and healthy balanced hormones, improve the appearance of your skin, help your body heal, and promote an overall sense of well-being.

Fats are satisfying, too, because they trigger the release of hormones that can help you feel full—which is one reason why you won't go hungry on the Galveston Diet. Fats are beneficial in other ways, too. For example, they help reverse insulin resistance, decrease the frequency of hot flashes, and curb the severity of night sweats.

In addition to good oils like olive oil, you can enjoy seeds and nuts as a fat source. Flax seeds, in particular, are rich in plant-based estrogens, especially lignans, which promote hormone regulation. They're also rich in omega-3 fatty acids, antioxidants, and fiber. Other seeds, like chia and hemp, are high in omega-3 fats.

Nuts are rich in the fats that are responsible for aiding the health of blood vessels and in hormone production. Additionally, they help lower cholesterol and regulate insulin levels while normalizing blood sugar.

Here is a comprehensive list of all the fats you can eat.

Galveston Diet—Approved Fats

Avocados
Avocado oil
Butter, preferably from grass-fed cows
Coconut flakes (in moderation)
Coconut flour (for use in recipes)
Coconut oil (in moderation)
Creamy dressing (for use in recipes)
Dairy fats (heavy cream, full-fat milk), if tolerated
Flaxseed oil
Ghee (clarified butter)
Hummus
Mayonnaise, preferably made with olive oil or avocado oil
MCT oil (in moderation)
Nuts, especially walnuts, almonds, pecans, macadamias; almond flour
Nut butters, sugar-free and free of added oils
Olive oil
Olives
Seed butters, sugar-free and free of added oils
Seeds, especially chia, flax, hemp, pumpkin, sunflower seeds
Sesame oil (in moderation)
Tahini (sesame seed butter)

Quality Proteins

Protein is to your body what wood is to your house and steel is to a skyscraper. It is the body's fundamental building material, and it plays a critical role in repair and maintenance. The Galveston Diet is thus a little higher in protein than many other plans.

If you've paid attention to nutritional advice in recent years, maybe you've encountered the pros and cons of eating more protein. Let me set the record straight: diets higher in protein have been unjustifiably criticized.

The truth is that women need more protein as they get older because their bodies tend to lose lean muscle and do less repair of old tissue. Much of this is due to the decline in estrogen, which is linked to losses in muscle mass and bone strength. To put it bluntly, protein is a lifesaver now. In a landmark study of women—the Women's Health Initiative—higher protein intake was associated with a 32 percent lower risk of frailty and with better physical function.

Further, protein also stabilizes blood sugar (helpful if you have mood swings). It influences the release of leptin and ghrelin, the hormones that regulate your appetite and food intake.

I recommend consuming a variety of protein: chicken, fish, lean meat, beans and legumes, dairy proteins, and more. Eggs are good, despite what we were once told. In fact, they are an inexpensive source of protein, and one of the best foods for balancing hunger and fat-storage hormones, because they have a positive impact on insulin and ghrelin. Eggs are rich in vitamin D, as well as in iron and B vitamins. Almost all the nutrients we need to feel our best and keep our bones strong are packaged in one small shell.

Fish is another rock star. Packed with inflammation-fighting omega-3 fats, the fattier fish such as wild-caught salmon, herring, mackerel, lake trout, and sardines stabilize your hunger hormones, leaving you feeling full for a longer period of time. On top of that, fatty fish are rich in vitamin D, which helps improve female testosterone levels. Getting these hormonal levels under control can positively address a woman's concerns about weight gain, fatigue, or depression. Fish can also keep the heart healthy and the skin and hair glowing.

Poultry and beef are excellent protein choices, too. They help promote the secretion of hormones such as leptin, which provides feelings of satiety. Animal proteins are also an important source of iron and vitamin B12.

Here's a rundown of the many protein types you can enjoy on this program.

Galveston Diet—Approved Proteins

Anchovies
Bacon, uncured, nitrate-free
Beef, lean cuts
Beef jerky, nitrate-free
Bison
Buffalo
Chicken
Collagen protein powder
Cornish hens
Duck
Eggs
Fish, wild-caught, especially salmon, trout, and tuna
Game such as venison
Legumes
Nitrate/nitrite free deli meats
Ostrich
Pork, lean cuts
Protein powder, limited ingredient, low sugar, low carbohydrate
Shellfish
Tofu
Turkey
Turkey bacon

Dairy Proteins

Unless you're lactose intolerant or can't digest dairy products, the Galveston Diet encourages some dairy. One of the main reasons is that the decline in estrogen levels during menopause can increase a woman's risk of fractures, and dairy foods are high in bone-building calcium.

The strength of your bones depends very much on adequate amounts of not only calcium but also vitamin D, also available from dairy protein.

Without these nutrients, your bones can slowly dissolve, becoming weak and prone to breaking. Thus, prevention is essential.

In one study that involved nearly 750 postmenopausal women, those who ate more dairy and animal protein had significantly higher bone density than those who ate less of the dairy and animal protein.

Dairy foods may also help you sleep better. A study reported that foods high in the amino acid glycine—widespread in milk and cheese, for example—promoted deeper sleep in perimenopausal and postmenopausal women.

Some dairy foods, especially yogurt, contain probiotics, which are beneficial bacteria. The probiotics can help boost the population of beneficial bacteria within the vagina and thus help prevent vaginal infections. They also reduce the symptoms of vaginal infections, such as vaginal discharge and odor, and are thus helpful for the treatment of infections.

Galveston Diet—Approved Vegetable Proteins

Almond milk/cheese/flour
Cashew milk/cheese
Chia seeds
Chickpeas/chickpea flour
Dried or canned beans
Edamame
Hemp hearts/milk
Lentils
Lupin beans
Nutritional Yeast
Seitan
Tempeh
Tofu

Hot Flash: 10 Surprising Benefits of Probiotics

When you think about probiotics like yogurt, gut health probably comes to mind. It's true that they help prevent and treat digestive conditions such as diarrhea, constipation, and inflammatory bowel diseases; and overall, they keep your gut microbiome—the trillions of bacteria in your gut—balanced and healthy. But although the many benefits of probiotics start in your gut, they don't end there. Probiotics also:

1. Help you lose weight and belly fat.
2. Improve some mental health conditions, such as depression, anxiety, and memory loss.
3. Keep your heart healthy.
4. Improve cholesterol levels and triglycerides.
5. Boost your immune system.
6. Maintain urogenital health.
7. Help your body manage blood sugar.
8. Strengthen bones and joints.
9. Protect against liver disease.
10. Help improve cancer outcomes.

There are lots of positives about dairy! Here's a list of foods you can include.

Galveston Diet—Approved Dairy Proteins

Cheddar
Cottage cheese, full-fat
Cream cheese
Feta cheese
Goat cheese
Greek yogurt, full-fat

Havarti
Heavy cream
Kefir, full fat
Monterey Jack
Mozzarella and other softer cheeses
Parmesan and other hard cheeses
Sour cream
Swiss

Carbohydrates

I want you to enjoy carbs—the good ones. Those are mainly the non-starchy carbs such as vegetables and some fruits, and the starchier carbs like sweet potatoes, fruits, and certain whole grains. All these foods are packed with vitamins, minerals, fiber, and antioxidants.

Stocking your fridge with leafy greens is important, too. Greens like spinach, kale, collard greens, and chard are loaded with antioxidants and can help prevent inflammation. Leafy greens can also help with hormones, especially estrogen metabolism. Additionally, they are high in fiber.

Broccoli, cabbage, cauliflower, kale, and Brussels sprouts are all part of the cruciferous vegetable family. Like leafy greens, these vegetables help process and remove excess estrogen from the body. One study revealed that eating broccoli lowered levels of a type of estrogen linked to breast cancer, while boosting an estrogen that protects against this disease.

Many of these high-quality carbs contain natural phytoestrogens. These are compounds in foods that act as weak estrogens in the body. Although there has been some controversy about including these in a diet, the most recent studies report they have health benefits for women in menopause. Foods that naturally contain phytoestrogens include soybeans, chickpeas, peanuts, flax seeds, berries, and green and black teas, among others.

Fruits are a natural way to calm a sweet tooth, and they are full of inflammation-fighting antioxidants. They are also high in water and fiber content, both of which fill you up without filling you out.

Galveston Diet—Approved Non-Starchy Vegetables

All leafy greens
Artichokes
Asparagus
Bamboo shoots
Bean sprouts
Beans, green or yellow (wax)
Beets
Bok choy
Broccoli
Broccolini
Brussels sprouts
Cabbage, all varieties
Carrots
Cauliflower
Celery
Cucumbers
Eggplant
Endive
Kimchi
Kohlrabi
Jicama
Mushrooms
Okra
Onions
Parsley
Peppers, all varieties and colors
Pickles
Radishes
Rutabaga
Sauerkraut
Scallions
Summer squash
Tomatoes
Watercress
Zucchini

Galveston Diet—Approved Starchy Vegetables

Edamame (soybeans)
Legumes, including lentils
Parsnips
Peas
Plantains
Potatoes
Turnips
Succotash (corn and lima beans)
Sweet potatoes (yams)
Winter squash

Galveston Diet—Approved Whole Grains

Amaranth (cooked in a similar way as rice or used as a flour)
Barley
Brown rice
Buckwheat (usually processed into groats, flour, or noodles)
Bulgur
Corn
Farro
Millet
Oats
Quinoa
Spelt (as cooked berries or flakes)
Wheat berries

Galveston Diet—Approved Fruits

Apples
Bananas
Blackberries
Blueberries
Cherries
Cranberries (fresh)
Grapefruit and other citrus fruits
Pears
Plums
Raspberries
Strawberries

Hot Flash: My Favorite Foods to Battle Hot Flashes

Up to 85 percent of menopausal women report hot flashes. These hot flashes can also occur in as many as 55 percent of women who are perimenopausal, and their incidence and severity can increase as the woman gets closer to menopause.

If you're experiencing hot flashes, you might find this statistic discouraging, but don't despair! Nutrition plays a huge role in combating hot flashes. Indeed, eating the Galveston Diet way can reduce them significantly. Here's a list of nutrients and foods that will put a lid on those overheating episodes.

Omega-3 fatty acids. Foods rich in these fats, such as salmon, tuna, walnuts, and flax seeds, can decrease the severity and frequency of hot flashes.

Vitamin E. Foods high in vitamin E, such as leafy greens, pumpkin and sunflower seeds, almonds, and red bell pepper, can help reduce hot flashes. Vitamin E is also a powerful antioxidant and is thought to help repair damaged cells in our bodies.

Soy foods. Soy-rich foods such as tofu and edamame may help alleviate hot flashes because they contain phytoestrogens. As a bonus, soy foods contain protein, fiber, and healthy fats.

Fruits and veggies. We know through research that women who consistently eat a diet rich in fruits and vegetables and who avoid sugar and processed foods have very few menopausal symptoms, such as hot flashes, weight gain, and the accumulation of visceral fat.

Fiber Up!

I've always been a major advocate for eating more fiber. From my work as a physician, I've known that people who consume the most fiber are the healthiest. Fortunately, you can increase your fiber intake easily on the Galveston Diet; over time, your efforts will pay off and you'll feel the benefits. That's because fiber does the following.

Controls appetite. Fiber helps slow down the delivery of nutrients to the gut and thus leaves you feeling full for longer, thereby suppressing your appetite. With less appetite, you may lose weight without even having to think about it. Fiber can also help reduce levels of the hunger hormone ghrelin.

Trims your waistline. If you've been doing a lot of crunches lately, but you're starting to lose faith that the bulge at your waist will ever shrink, you need to up your fiber intake, especially the soluble type. Some evidence indicates that the weight-loss effects of this fiber specifically target belly fat.

Fiber in general can help you shed pounds in other ways, too. For instance, it takes a long time to chew most high-fiber foods. This slows down the process of eating, allowing the satiety signals to reach your brain before you've overeaten. Fiber may also reduce the amount of calories your body absorbs from other foods you eat.

Regulates blood sugar and insulin. A well-demonstrated benefit of fiber is its effect on blood-sugar levels and insulin requirements. Lots of research with healthy subjects and people with diabetes have shown that when fiber is eaten along with carbohydrates, the blood levels of carbohydrates and insulin don't rise as high as when carbs are eaten without fiber.

Reduces breast cancer risk. A statistical review of studies on the subject found that women who followed fiber-rich diets could reduce their risk of breast cancer by 12 percent. How exactly does fiber pull this off? Fiber does the following:

- Decreases the level of excess estrogen in the blood circulation.
- Combines with harmful and carcinogenic substances in the gut and, like a broom, sweeps through your digestive system and ushers them out of your body.
- Promotes the growth of healthy bacteria in the gut and inhibits the growth of bad bacteria—a process that interferes with the production of carcinogens and promotes their decomposition in the gut.
- Improves the ingestion of bad bacteria by macrophages, the white blood cells that make up part of your immune system.
- Promotes short-chain fatty acids (SCFAs), which help fend off the growth of tumor cells.

You should eat at least 25 grams of fiber a day—more if you can. This isn't as tough as it seems if you eat a lot of veggies and some fruit each day.

Galveston Diet Foods with the Most Fiber

Food Source	Serving Size	Grams of Fiber
Artichoke	1 medium, cooked	10
Avocado	1 cup diced	10
Peas	1 cup cooked	9
Winter squash	1 cup cooked	9
Berries, fresh	1 cup	8
Lentils	1/2 cup cooked	8
Black beans	1/2 cup cooked	7.5
Garbanzo beans	1/2 cup cooked	6
Parsnips	1 cup cooked	6
Pear, with skin	1 medium	5.5
Broccoli	1 cup cooked	5
Collard greens	1 cup cooked	5
Apple, with skin	1 medium	4.3
Brussels sprouts	1 cup cooked	4
Green beans	1 cup cooked	4
Okra	1 cup cooked	4
Potato	1 medium, cooked	4
Sweet potato	1 medium, cooked	4
Bulgur wheat	1/2 cup cooked	4
Spelt	1/2 cup cooked	3.8
Corn kernels	1/2 cup cooked	3.5
Cherries, fresh	1 cup	3.2
Kale	1 cup cooked	3
Barley	1/2 cup cooked	3

Increase Intake of Magnesium

One mineral you get a lot of on the Galveston Diet is magnesium. This important but underappreciated mineral is key to women's health. It is involved in hundreds of biochemical reactions throughout the body and is critical to energy stores and muscle and nerve function. It is estimated that 50 percent of women don't get enough of it in their diet. What's more, as you get older and experience menopause, magnesium becomes particularly important for good health; it may even help reduce menopause symptoms and conditions. Magnesium does the following.

Keeps bones strong. Approximately 60 percent of a person's magnesium is stored in the bones, so it plays a big role in preventing osteoporosis (along with calcium). With the declining levels of estrogen during menopause, the bones start breaking down at a faster rate than they are rebuilt, leading to weakened, porous bones. Magnesium helps prevent this breakdown because it helps increase the calcification of the bone matrix.

What's more, magnesium helps decrease inflammation, which weakens bones over time.

Prevents insulin resistance and diabetes. Low amounts of magnesium can make you vulnerable to these conditions, which you don't want because they can bring on many other complications.

Researchers have known for a long time that diabetes is linked to a magnesium deficiency. That is, people with diabetes are thought to have a peculiar defect in the metabolism of magnesium. Fortunately, including fairly low doses of magnesium in your diet can help prevent diabetic complications and can intervene in the course of the disease itself.

Guards heart health. Magnesium seems to protect the heart in several different ways: it prevents abnormal heart rhythms, deters the formation of blood clots, and regulates blood pressure.

One reason it is so favorable for the heart is that magnesium-rich foods are a significant source of antioxidants, healthy fats, protein, and fiber, all of which benefit heart health. In one study of nearly 4,000 postmenopausal women, high magnesium levels were associated with lower inflammatory markers related to heart disease, indicating better heart health.

Enhances sleep. Up to 60 percent of menopausal women experience insomnia or have difficulty sleeping. Those who do nod off may have poor sleep quality. Magnesium can help here, too, because it appears to promote sleep by regulating the body's circadian rhythms (known as the body's natural clock) and increasing muscle relaxation.

One small study of 46 older adults found that supplementing with 500 mg of magnesium daily led to a significant increase in sleep duration, sleep quality, and the production of melatonin (a sleep hormone), while no improvements were seen in the control group.

Lifts your mood. If you're suffering from depression and don't want to take antidepressants, reach for some magnesium. The reason magnesium may chase away the blues is its positive impact on brain function, mood regulation, and stress response—all of which may affect the progression and onset of depression.

Boosts fat burn. We don't commonly think of magnesium as being a fat burner, but it does help with weight loss. Emerging research has found that it reduces insulin resistance. This is a condition in which you have too much insulin and it doesn't do its job properly; the result is that your body can't burn fat as efficiently, including stubborn belly fat. Insulin resistance can also increase cravings for carbohydrate-rich snacks. So, magnesium may be helpful for regulating blood sugar and insulin levels in people who are overweight or obese. Magnesium also helps resolve bloating and water retention.

Goes beyond menopause. Magnesium helps prevent and treat many diseases, especially those associated with a short supply of it. This includes Alzheimer's disease, insulin resistance, type 2 diabetes, high blood pressure, cardiovascular disease, and migraines.

Women need 310 to 320 mg of magnesium daily. See the following chart for sources of magnesium.

n Diet Foods with the Most Magnesium

Food Source	Serving Size	Milligrams
eafy greens	1 cup cooked	156
Pumpkin seeds	1 ounce (2 tablespoons)	150
Salmon	1 fillet cooked	106
Mackerel	1 small fillet cooked	97
Almonds	1 ounce (2 tablespoons)	80
Cashews	1 ounce (2 tablespoons)	72
Chocolate, dark	1-ounce piece	64
Quinoa	1/2 cup cooked	60
Avocado	1 medium	58
Tofu	3 1/2-ounce square, cooked	53
Edamame	1/2 cup cooked	50
Flax seeds	1 ounce (2 tablespoons)	40
Black beans	1/2 cup cooked	40
Lima beans	1/2 cup cooked	40

Boost Your Omega-3 Fatty Acids

The benefits of omega-3 fats in menopause are considerable, which is why I've talked a great deal about them in this book. They are plentiful in the Galveston Diet because these fats do the following.

Reverse that middle-age spread. As mentioned earlier, EPA and DHA are the omega-3 fatty acids found primarily in fatty fish. Both can actually reduce body fat, particularly in the belly. Researchers in China did a statistical analysis of seven studies involving omega-3 fats and overweight adults, and they concluded that supplementation with omega-3s produced a significant reduction in waist circumference.

Curb hunger. In a study of 232 overweight and obese volunteers, researchers put the subjects (who were in the last two weeks of an eight-week weight-loss plan) on either high or low doses of omega-3s. Those taking the high doses reported feeling fuller and less hungry two hours after their meal than did those who took the lower doses of omega-3s.

Reduce triglycerides. As you enter midlife, your triglyceride levels may soar. And as those triglyceride levels rise, unfortunately the levels of good-type HDL cholesterol fall, dramatically increasing your risk of heart disease.

Postmenopausal women may have higher triglyceride concentrations than premenopausal women, exposing them to increased risk of heart disease. Omega-3 fatty acids are a must here. They help lower triglycerides, in conjunction with a diet very low in sugar and refined carbs.

Ease menopause-related joint pain. Omega-3 fats help discourage the formation of hormone-like agents called prostaglandins. These agents can trigger inflammation that can harm your joints. Omega-3 fats come to the rescue here. They powerfully fight inflammation, and in the process they help relieve joint pain and stiffness in menopause. In fact, these fats work in a similar way as non-steroidal anti-inflammatory drugs (NSAIDs).

Help with the blues. Women are twice as likely to suffer from depression as men, and the risk is even greater following menopause. Irritability and sadness are common emotional symptoms of menopause, but omega-3 fats may ease these symptoms by restoring structural integrity to the brain cells that are critical in performing cognitive functions.

Support bone health. Eating more omega-3 acids has been found to boost bone mineral content and help prevent osteoporosis. So, make these fats an essential part of your diet.

Get your sexual mojo back. Omega-3 fats help lubricate your body in general, therefore helping with dryness of the vagina—a common symptom of perimenopause, menopause, and postmenopause.

Most women need at least 2 grams of omega-3 fats daily. See the following chart for sources and serving sizes.

Galveston Diet Foods with the Most Omega-3 Fats

Food	Serving Size	Milligrams
Flaxseed oil	1 tablespoon	7,260
Chia seeds	2 tablespoons	5,060
Salmon	3 1/2 ounces cooked	4,123
Mackerel	3 1/2 ounces cooked	4,107
Walnuts, chopped	2 tablespoons	2,570
Flax seeds	1 tablespoon	2,350
Sardines	3 1/2-ounce can	1,480
Hemp seeds	1 tablespoon	1,000
Anchovies	2-ounce can	951
Herring, fresh or canned	3 1/2 ounces	946
Soybeans	1/2 cup cooked	670
Tofu, firm	3 1/2-ounce square	495
Oysters	6, shucked raw	370
Winter squash	1 cup cooked	332
Omega-3 enriched eggs	1 egg, large	225
Spinach	1 cup cooked	166

Ease Your Menopause Issues with Vitamin D

I can't say enough good things about vitamin D. Technically a hormone rather than a vitamin, vitamin D shines for its health benefits, particularly in the proper functioning of your heart, lungs, blood vessels, and immune system. As for menopause issues, vitamin D can help in the following ways.

Supports weight loss. As a fat burner, vitamin D works in three key ways. First, when your vitamin D levels are good, your body manufactures more leptin, the hormone that tells your brain that you're full and to stop eating. Second, with an ample supply of this vitamin, your fat cells resist making and storing fat. Third, vitamin D interacts with calcium to halt the overproduction of cortisol, the notorious stress hormone that, when chronically elevated, triggers the storage of belly fat.

Boosts muscle strength. The case for getting enough vitamin D is so persuasive that it goes right down to your muscle strength and mass, which decline with age. A recent study documented that this vitamin can significantly increase muscle strength and reduce the loss of body muscle mass in women as late as 12 or more years after menopause.

In this clinical trial, 160 Brazilian postmenopausal women were randomized into two groups: a group receiving 1,000 units of vitamin D daily and a placebo group. The researchers found at the end of the 9-month study that the women who received the vitamin supplements showed an increase of more than 25 percent in muscle strength. Those in the control group lost an average of 6.8 percent of muscle mass. The women in that group were also nearly twice as likely to fall.

Helps with depression. Research has shown that vitamin D might play an important role in regulating mood and decreasing the risk of depression. Published in *Depression and Anxiety* in 2020, a review of 7,534 people found that those experiencing negative emotions who received vitamin D supplements noticed an improvement in symptoms. The study also concluded that vitamin D supplementation may help people with depression who also have a vitamin D deficiency.

Resolves fatigue. Fatigue is a common menopause complaint, especially in the early stages of menopause as the body adjusts to its fluctuating hormones. One study from 2015 involving female nurses found a strong connection between low vitamin D levels and self-reported fatigue. What's more, 89 percent of the participants were deficient in this vitamin.

Reboots your bones. Poor bone mineral density is a sign that your bones are weakening owing to the loss of calcium and other minerals. This condition places older adults, especially women, at a higher risk of fractures. Regularly getting sufficient vitamin D and calcium at the same time helps your body maximize absorption of calcium, leading to stronger bones.

Cuts breast cancer risk. It has been demonstrated that treating breast cancer cells with vitamin D stops the growth and spread of breast cancer cells and initiates a process that encourages the death of those cells.

Women ages 19 to 50 should get 600 international units (IUs) of vitamin D daily as a minimum for maintenance; women over 50 should get 800 IUs. Although it's possible to do this with a diet rich in vitamin D, it is also a good idea to take a supplement. This will ensure that you're getting the appropriate amount each day.

The following chart lists the foods that are good sources of vitamin D.

Galveston Diet Foods with the Most Vitamin D

Food	Serving Size	IUs
Mushrooms (D2)	3 1/2 ounces cooked	2,300
Salmon, wild-caught	3 1/2 ounces cooked	1,300
Sardines	3 1/2-ounce can	270
Tuna	3 1/2-ounce can	268
Herring, fresh or canned	3 1/2 ounces	216
Oatmeal	1/2 cup cooked	150
Milk	1 cup	100
Yogurt	3/4 cup	100
Almond milk	1 cup	100
Cheese, hard	1 slice or 1 ounce, depending on the cheese	40
Egg yolk	1 large	37

Drink Up!

I recommend you get at least 64 ounces (8 cups) of water a day. Water is a vital nutrient, but it's also one of our most neglected ones. Water just has so many benefits, ranging from heart health to brain function, to the elimination of toxins from the body. For women, it helps prevent dryness symptoms (like vaginal and skin dryness, common with menopause), and bloating (which can come with hormonal changes). Overall, water lubricates our bodies.

Here's the red flag: avoid store-bought flavored waters; they are almost always loaded with sugar and artificial additives. If plain water doesn't appeal to you, infuse your own with fruits, herbs, or veggies like sliced cucumbers. It's quick and easy to do and is a great way to use these foods.

Sugar Alternatives

Stevia and erythritol (with or without monk fruit) are the only acceptable sugar alternatives known to not cause a spike in your insulin or glucose.

Many women ask me if these sugar alternatives can be used during the fasting period. Personally, I do not consume anything sweet while fasting, but the jury is still out on whether it affects fasting or not. Some scientists believe that when the sweet receptors of the digestive tract are stimulated by these substances, insulin is released, negating some of the benefits of fasting.

Swerve sweetener is a popular brand of erythritol blend, available in both confectioners' and granular form.

The Joy of Change

The Galveston Diet has proved to be an extremely effective program for resolving the symptoms and illnesses associated with midlife. Recently, I was moved by the healing stories of two participants, Bonnie and Donna, both of whom had a cluster of health problems.

Bonnie, who began the program in 2019, had a fatty liver, diabetes, abnormal cholesterol, and atrial fibrillation (also referred to as a-fib, which is an irregular and often very rapid heart rhythm, or arrhythmia, that can lead to blood clots in the heart). What happened after she was well into the program was near miraculous. "I had a health transformation. I no longer have a fatty liver. My cholesterol levels are within the normal ranges. I'm no longer diabetic. I haven't had an a-fib episode in a year. I've lost 42 pounds since starting the program."

Her cardiologist added, "Taking control of [her] health and diet has directly affected [her] heart health." Her primary care physician weighed in, too: "With [her] diet change, [she] has dodged some bullets."

Donna, age 73, was taking eight medications for various conditions, including high blood pressure, high blood sugar, and high cholesterol. After starting the Galveston Diet in February 2020, she reported: "Although weight loss was not my initial concern, I lost a total of 24 pounds and many inches. But what I'm most proud of is that my A1c [an indicator of diabetes] dropped from 7.2 to a more normal 5.9. My blood pressure is within a normal range, and my total cholesterol is 135. I'm now taking only two medications."

These stories are the norm for program participants, not the exception. So, eat certain foods according to the diet, not just because they will help you lose pounds and inches but also because they are both healthful and healing—and will produce life-transforming results for you.

As I've said repeatedly, what you eat every day on the Galveston Diet has a profound and everlasting impact on your health, weight, and longevity. Foods are concoctions of some awesome nutrients that, when consumed, enter your cells, improving their activity and function. What you give your cells through your food choices can make your body so strong that you can boost your prospects for living an amazingly long and healthy life.

CHAPTER 8

Putting It All Together: The Meal Plans and Shopping Lists

Welcome to the Galveston Diet meal plans! To get started on this new way of eating, I provide here four weeks of conventional menus and two weeks of vegetarian menus—with no calculations required. All these meals have ample portions of healthy fats, lean protein, and good carbohydrates, in the proper ratios. These meals also contribute fiber, magnesium, omega-3 fatty acids, vitamin D, and other important nutrients that support midlife health. Each meal is proportioned just right to satisfy your hunger and help you feel full afterwards. The recipes for these meal plans are included in Chapter 9.

As you see in the pages that follow, the daily plans include two meals and two snacks a day (to be eaten within your eating window). Each daily plan is followed by a macronutrient ratio analysis so you can see the balance and track how you'll get close to the recommended 70/20/10 proportion each day. Remember, you won't be counting calories on this program; focus on macronutrient ratios instead.

Every week of plans is followed with a shopping list so you can plan your week's meals and buy the foods you'll need. The lists are based on using the meal plans as written, but you can, of course, adapt them to your needs, to other recipes you want to include, and to how many people you'll be cooking for.

Having a detailed shopping list is essential for sticking to the week's meal plan, especially in these early weeks when you are getting used to this new eating style. Knowing what to eat, how much to eat, and when to eat, and having the ingredients readily available to prepare the meals as designed, is one of the most important aspects of this program.

The key to good meal prep is to have a few basic foods that you can prepare and cook ahead, divide into batches, and then use in many different ways during the week. Take that extra time to prepare for the week ahead, and you'll be rewarded with the following:

Better nutrition. Following meal plans means you have control of the nutrition, ingredients, and portions that you eat during the week. This saves time and eliminates many decisions that might otherwise jeopardize your waistline.

Better metabolism. You'll be prepared at snack time when that hunger strikes because you'll have something nourishing and nutritious—snacks that will fill you up, lower any inflammation, and help burn fat.

Wiser purchasing. Planning and prepping your meals will save you money. Skip the $15 each weekday you spend on a takeout salad covered in croutons and drenched with some unknown dressing (often with preservatives and chemicals), and you'll save $75. Use that money to splurge on a massage or facial instead.

To best make use of the meal plans, try following some of these meal prep suggestions:

1. **Plan ahead.** Decide what meals you'll focus on for the week and how many meals you'll need to prepare. Keep a running inventory

of what's in your fridge, freezer, and pantry, and note the basic items you are running low on.

2. **Make up your shopping list before you go to the grocery store.** It's preferable to bring your market list to the store, so you know exactly what you need to purchase. Once you get there, stick to the outer aisles as much as possible, as that's where you'll find the fresh food, fruit, and vegetables. Stock up on pantry basics, too, such as olive oils in different flavors, a variety of nuts and seeds, and various spices and condiments. And don't forget about your local farmers' market; it is a great source of very fresh fruits and vegetables in season. But if you're short on time, most markets have a "click list" or online shop, where you can purchase your items at home and then you can just pick up the packages or have them delivered. This way you avoid the checkout line.
3. **Read over the recipes for the week.** If your cooking skills are minimal, start with the easier recipes or those similar to what you've prepared before and are confident about making. You can then ease into other, less familiar preparations, learning as you go and exploring new taste combinations. If you're not familiar with using an outdoor grill, opt for a grill pan on the stove or another cooking method before you attempt to grill meat or vegetables outside.
4. **Ensure your meals have variety.** If you've planned the protein foundation for your meal, sometimes introduce different vegetables, fruits, and healthy fats to ensure you're getting a variety of micronutrients. Go for colorful foods, and "eat the rainbow."
5. **Have food storage containers handy.** Glass is always best for taking food from the fridge to the microwave, but plastic containers may be more practical for packing lunch boxes. Consider packaging for your snacks as well. Zipper-topped plastic bags are great for small items such as nuts and seeds.
6. **Use efficiency without sacrificing quality.** In your food purchases, stock up on frozen vegetables when they are on sale, consider spending a few cents more for pre-cut vegetables to save prep

time, and purchase already trimmed or pre-cooked lean proteins for greater convenience. But always read the labels or ask what ingredients were used in the preparation or any prepared foods.

7. **Lighten the mood.** When you're prepping or cooking your meals, perhaps listen to your favorite podcast, audio book, or soundtrack—or save your guilty pleasure TV show to watch while you're in the kitchen.

Meals are not always on-the-spot cooking; they can be prepped and cooked in a variety of ways. Explore these two styles of meal prep:

Make-ahead meals. These are full meals cooked hours in advance, then refrigerated and reheated at mealtime. This is a helpful method for handling dinner meals, especially when feeding a family.

Batch cooking. Make a large batch of a recipe and then split it into individual portions and freeze them for future use. For example, if you're making a pot of chili, portion out a serving or two and place it in the fridge, then portion the rest into individual servings, place in storage containers, label with the date, and freeze for future enjoyment.

Individual portions. Prepare a recipe and store it in grab-and-go small portions that can be taken out of the refrigerator and quickly heated or enjoyed cold. This is a great option for breakfast meals.

The Conventional Menus: Week 1

DAY 1

MEAL 1: MARY CLAIRE'S PARFAIT (PAGE 173)

Snack 1: Celery Sticks with Almond Butter (page 207)

MEAL 2: MEATLOAF WITH CAULIFLOWER MASH (PAGE 198)

Snack 2: Pecans and Dark Chocolate (page 216)

Macros: Fat: 70%, Protein: 20%, Net Carbs: 10%, Fiber: 23g

DAY 2

MEAL 1: EGG SCRAMBLE (PAGE 174)

Snack 1: Caprese Bites (page 207)

MEAL 2: GRILLED CHICKEN SALAD (PAGE 189)

Snack 2: Chia Pudding (page 221)

Macros: Fat: 71%, Protein: 21%, Net Carbs: 8%, Fiber: 29g

DAY 3

MEAL 1: MEATLOAF WITH CAULIFLOWER MASH (FROM DAY 1)

Snack 1: Avocado Crisps (page 209)

MEAL 2: BAKED SALMON WITH GRILLED SUMMER SQUASH (PAGE 193)

Snack 2: Chia Pudding (page 221)

Macros: Fat: 70%, Protein: 23%, Net Carbs: 7%, Fiber: 24g

DAY 4

MEAL 1: MARY CLAIRE'S PARFAIT (PAGE 173)

Snack 1: Easy Guacamole (page 211) with bell pepper strips

MEAL 2: GRILLED CHICKEN SALAD (FROM DAY 2)

Snack 2: Raspberries with Pecans (page 216)

Macros: Fat: 70%, Protein: 21%, Net Carbs: 9%, Fiber: 31g

DAY 5

MEAL 1: TUNA SALAD WITH SNACKY SIDE SALAD (PAGE 179)

Snack 1: Easy Guacamole (from day 4) with baby carrots

MEAL 2: BAKED SALMON WITH GRILLED SUMMER SQUASH (FROM DAY 3)

Snack 2: Raspberry-Flax Muffin (page 224)

Macros: Fat: 74%, Protein: 18%, Net Carbs: 8%, Fiber: 32g

DAY 6

MEAL 1: TUNA SALAD WITH SNACKY SIDE SALAD (PAGE 179)

Snack 1: Carrots and Celery with Flax Seed and Almond Butter (page 207)

MEAL 2: CHICKEN TACO SALAD (PAGE 182)

Snack 2: Raspberry-Flax Muffin (page 224)

Macros: Fat: 73%, Protein: 19%, Net Carbs: 8%, Fiber: 25g

DAY 7

MEAL 1: EGG SCRAMBLE (PAGE 174)

Snack 1: Caprese Bites (page 207)

MEAL 2: MEATLOAF WITH CAULIFLOWER MASH (FROM DAY 1)

Snack 2: Pecans with Berries and Coconut (page 215)

Macros: Fat: 66%, Protein: 17%, Net Carbs: 15%, Fiber: 25g

General Guidelines for Using the Shopping Lists

As you set out to shop for your first week of eating the Galveston Diet way, you'll want to do a general shopping for pantry and other staples that you will use for the entire program. See the list that follows for the staples you'll use frequently when eating on the Galveston Diet. Then, follow the weekly shopping lists for the fresh foods and other particulars you'll need each week.

The food quantities included in each week's shopping list are closest to the quantity you will need for that week's recipes. When possible, I've rounded off the amount to a market size, but I often give the actual quantity needed so that you can be assured you have the right amount.

Also, the quantities listed are for making the yields as noted in the recipes. The assumption is that you are cooking mostly for yourself, and the higher yields indicate that you'll be eating that recipe more than once during the week. But if you are cooking for others as well, you will need to increase your grocery purchases (and/or repeat making the dish) to correspond with the larger number of portions you need. Carefully check the recipe yields and build your shopping list around those meals. Remember, the shopping lists are a general guideline for what you'll need during the week; you may have on hand ingredients from a previous week, or you may decide not to make a particular recipe.

Pantry Staples

Spices, Seasonings, and Flavorings

- ☐ Almond extract
- ☐ Black pepper, ground
- ☐ Cayenne pepper
- ☐ Chili powder
- ☐ Cinnamon, ground
- ☐ Cumin, ground
- ☐ Curry powder
- ☐ "Everything bagel" seasoning
- ☐ Garlic powder
- ☐ Garlic salt
- ☐ Italian seasoning
- ☐ Mustard, stone-ground
- ☐ Nutmeg, ground
- ☐ Onion powder
- ☐ Oregano, dried
- ☐ Paprika, smoked and sweet
- ☐ Pumpkin pie spice
- ☐ Red pepper flakes
- ☐ Salt: kosher, sea salt, and table salt
- ☐ Turmeric, ground
- ☐ Vanilla bean paste
- ☐ Vanilla extract
- ☐ White pepper, ground

Oils and Fats

- ☐ Avocado oil
- ☐ Butter: salted and unsalted
- ☐ Coconut oil
- ☐ Ghee (clarified butter)
- ☐ Mayonnaise: regular (no added sugar), avocado oil mayo, olive oil mayo
- ☐ Olive oil
- ☐ Ranch dressing
- ☐ Toasted sesame oil

Nuts and Seeds

- [ ] Almonds: slivered and whole
- [ ] Chia seeds
- [ ] Coconut flakes, unsweetened
- [ ] Flaxseed, ground
- [ ] Hemp hearts
- [ ] Macadamia nuts: whole and halved
- [ ] Mixed nuts
- [ ] Peanuts: roasted and salted
- [ ] Pecans
- [ ] Pumpkin seeds
- [ ] Sesame seeds: black and white
- [ ] Sunflower seeds
- [ ] Walnuts

Condiments

- [ ] Primal Kitchen BBQ sauce
- [ ] Spicy brown mustard
- [ ] Sriracha or other hot sauce
- [ ] Tamari or soy sauce

Miscellaneous

- [ ] Almond butter, unsweetened
- [ ] Almond flour
- [ ] Apple butter
- [ ] Baking powder
- [ ] Cacao powder
- [ ] Coconut flour
- [ ] Coconut milk, unsweetened
- [ ] Cocoa powder, unsweetened
- [ ] Collagen powder
- [ ] Honey
- [ ] Maple syrup
- [ ] MCT powder
- [ ] Oat flour
- [ ] Peanut butter, no sugar added
- [ ] Vinegar: red wine, rice wine, balsamic, apple cider
- [ ] Sweeteners: stevia, monk fruit (with or without erythritol), Swerve

Shopping List for Week 1

Note: Amounts given here indicate the quantities you need for the week's recipes; they are not always indicative of the quantities in which the items are commonly sold.

Proteins

Beef, ground, $1^1/_2$ pounds lean, grass-fed
Chicken, 1 pound boneless, skinless breasts
Chicken, pre-cooked, 1 breast (about 8 ounces)
Salmon, 3-pound fillet
Eggs, 7 large
Mozzarella balls, whole-milk, 1 (8-ounce) package
Yogurt, plain full-fat Greek (such as Fage), 1 (16-ounce) container
Tuna, 2 (2-ounce) cans, packed in water

Vegetables

Carrots, baby, small package (10 ounces)
Carrots, 2 medium
Cauliflower, 1 large head
Celery, 1 stalk
Cherry tomatoes, 2 pints
Garlic bulb, 1
Onion, 1 medium white or yellow
Onion, 1 medium red
Romaine lettuce, 1 head
Tomato, 1 large Roma (plum)
Tomatoes, 1 to 2 ripe round
Spinach, 1 (10-ounce) bag
Summer squash, 1 medium yellow
Zucchini, 1 medium
Assorted raw veggies for dipping
Mixed salad greens, 1 bag

Fresh Herbs

Basil
Cilantro
Parsley

Fruits

Avocados, 4 medium

Blueberries, 1/2 pint

Lemons, 6 medium

Raspberries, 1/2 pint

Strawberries, 1 pint

Miscellaneous

(Small containers/packages of each)

Coconut milk, unsweetened

Parmesan cheese, pre-grated

Heavy cream

Sour cream

Dark chocolate chips, sugar-free

Tomato sauce, canned or jarred, no sugar added

Week 2

DAY 1

MEAL 1: ROASTED TOMATO BISQUE (PAGE 182)

Snack 1: Everything-Bagel Cucumber Bites (page 210)

MEAL 2: PORTOBELLO PIZZAS (PAGE 190)

Snack 2: Blueberry Pie Smoothie (page 218)

Macros: Fat: 72%, Protein: 16%, Net Carbs: 12%, Fiber: 28g

DAY 2

MEAL 1: TGD COBB SALAD (PAGE 179)

Snack 1: Fresh blueberries

MEAL 2: CHEESEBURGER LETTUCE SLIDERS (PAGE 191)

Snack 2: Chocolate-Cinnamon Apple Bites (page 224)

Macros: Fat: 66%, Protein: 24%, Net Carbs: 10%, Fiber: 21g

DAY 3

MEAL 1: ROASTED TOMATO BISQUE (FROM DAY 1)

Snack 1: Chocolate-Cinnamon Apple Bites (from day 2)

MEAL 2: TGD COBB SALAD (FROM DAY 2)

Snack 2: Tropical Berries (page 216)

Macros: Fat: 70%, Protein: 23%, Net Carbs: 7%, Fiber: 24g

DAY 4

MEAL 1: CHICKEN AND BLT WRAP (PAGE 178)

Snack 1: Herbed White Bean Dip (page 212) with cucumber slices

MEAL 2: CHEESEBURGER LETTUCE SLIDERS (FROM DAY 2)

Snack 2: Chocolate-Cinnamon Apple Bites (page 224)

Macros: Fat: 70%, Protein: 19%, Net Carbs: 11%, Fiber: 21g

DAY 5

MEAL 1: PORTOBELLO PIZZAS (PAGE 190)

Snack 1: Chocolate Peanut Butter Yogurt (page 223)

MEAL 2: CHICKEN AND BLT WRAP (FROM DAY 4)

Snack 2: Apple and mixed nuts

Macros: Fat: 67%, Protein: 20%, Net Carbs: 13%, Fiber: 25g

DAY 6

MEAL 1: AVOCADO "FOR LIFE" TOAST (PAGE 175)

Snack 1: Herbed White Bean Dip (from day 4) with cucumber slices

MEAL 2: SESAME GINGER PORK WITH GREEN BEANS (PAGE 183)

Snack 2: Coconut and Walnut Chia Pudding (page 222)

Macros: Fat: 68%, Protein: 18%, Net Carbs: 14%, Fiber: 34g

DAY 7

MEAL 1: SESAME GINGER PORK WITH GREEN BEANS (FROM DAY 6)

Snack 1: Cheese and Walnuts (page 209)

MEAL 2: GRILLED SHRIMP WITH BROILED TOMATO BITES (PAGE 194)

Snack 2: Chocolate–Peanut Butter Mug Cake (page 225)

Macros: Fat: 74%, Protein: 20%, Net Carbs: 6%, Fiber: 27g

Shopping List for Week 2

Proteins

Beef, ground, 6 ounces grass-fed, 90% lean
Chicken, 1 skinless, boneless breast (about 6 ounces)
Chicken, rotisserie-cooked, 1 to 2 breasts (12 ounces)
Eggs, 1 dozen large
Pork, boneless loin, 1 (8-ounce) piece
Turkey bacon, 1 pound
Shrimp, large, 1 pound
Yogurt, plain full-fat Greek, 1 (5.3-ounce) container

Vegetables

Cucumbers, 2 medium
Garlic, 10 cloves (1 head)
Green beans, fresh, 8 ounces
Mushrooms, portobello caps, 8
Onion, 1 medium red
Onion, 1 medium white or yellow
Romaine lettuce, 1 large head
Tomatoes, cherry, 1 pint
Tomatoes, grape, 1 pint
Tomatoes, Roma (plum), 8 medium
Tomatoes, 1 to 2 ripe round

Spinach, 1 (10-ounce) bag
2 (15-ounce) cans cannellini beans
Dill pickles, 1 (18-ounce) jar

Fresh Herbs
Basil
Dill
Ginger
Parsley

Fruits
Apple, 1
Avocados, 3 medium
Blueberries, 1/2 pint
Lemons, 2 medium
Raspberries, 1/2 pint

Miscellaneous
Cheddar cheese, pre-grated, 1 (9-ounce) package
Cheese sticks, small package
Chicken broth, 1 (16-ounce) can
Chocolate chips, sugar-free dark, 1 ounce
Coconut milk, unsweetened full-fat, 1 (15-ounce) can
Cream cheese, 1 (4-ounce) package
Mozzarella cheese, pre-shredded, 1 (2-ounce) package (about 1/2 cup)
Parmesan cheese, pre-grated, 1 (1-ounce) package (about 1/4 cup)
Sprouted-grain bread (such as Food For Life)

Week 3

DAY 1

MEAL 1: BELL PEPPERS STUFFED WITH TURKEY AND CAULIFLOWER RICE (PAGE 184)

Snack 1: Marinated Olives, Chickpeas, and Vegetables with Thyme and Dill (page 213)

MEAL 2: SHRIMP AND ASPARAGUS (PAGE 185)

Snack 2: Aloha Avocado (page 208)

Macros: Fat: 69%, Protein: 20%, Net Carbs: 11%, Fiber: 25g

DAY 2

MEAL 1: SHRIMP AND ASPARAGUS (FROM DAY 1)

Snack 1: Aloha Avocado (from day 1)

MEAL 2: SIRLOIN, SPINACH, AND BLUE CHEESE SALAD WITH PECANS (PAGE 196)

Snack 2: Marinated Olives, Chickpeas, and Vegetables with Thyme and Dill (from day 1)

Macros: Fat: 71%, Protein: 19%, Net Carbs: 10%, Fiber: 26g

DAY 3

MEAL 1: BELL PEPPERS STUFFED WITH TURKEY AND CAULIFLOWER RICE (FROM DAY 1)

Snack 1: Apple Clusters (page 208)

MEAL 2: GRILLED STEAK WITH CREAMED SPINACH AND MUSHROOMS (PAGE 199)

Snack 2: Veggie Slices with Italian Mayo Dip (page 212)

Macros: Fat: 65%, Protein: 22%, Net Carbs: 13%, Fiber: 22g

DAY 4

MEAL 1: SIRLOIN, SPINACH, AND BLUE CHEESE SALAD WITH PECANS (FROM DAY 2)

Snack 1: Marinated Olives, Chickpeas, and Vegetables with Thyme and Dill (from day 1)

MEAL 2: BELL PEPPERS STUFFED WITH TURKEY AND CAULIFLOWER RICE (FROM DAY 1)

Snack 2: Aloha Avocado (from day 1)

Macros: Fat: 70%, Protein: 21%, Net Carbs: 9%, Fiber: 24g

DAY 5

MEAL 1: BELL PEPPERS STUFFED WITH TURKEY AND CAULIFLOWER RICE (FROM DAY 1)

Snack 1: Aloha Avocado (from day 1)

MEAL 2: BROCCOLI AND CHEESE CHICKEN BAKE (PAGE 196), PLUS 2 TABLESPOONS GROUND FLAXSEED

Snack 2: Nutty Berry Bowl (page 216)

Macros: Fat: 69%, Protein: 24%, Net Carbs: 7%, Fiber: 25g

DAY 6

MEAL 1: COTTAGE CHEESE OMELET (PAGE 174)

Snack 1: Veggie Slices with Italian Mayo Dip (from day 3)

MEAL 2: BROCCOLI AND CHEESE CHICKEN BAKE (FROM DAY 5), PLUS 2 TABLESPOONS GROUND FLAXSEED AND SNACKY SIDE SALAD (PAGE 179)

Snack 2: Mixed Berry Smoothie (page 219)

Macros: Fat: 66%, Protein: 22%, Net Carbs: 13%, Fiber: 27g

DAY 7

MEAL 1: POACHED EGGS WITH CABBAGE HASH BROWNS (PAGE 175) AND AVOCADO HALF

Snack 1: Mary Claire's Parfait (page 173) blended to a smoothie

MEAL 2: TUNA SALAD OVER MIXED GREENS (PAGE 183)

Snack 2: Herbed Cottage Cheese Dip with Cucumber (page 212)

Macros: Fat: 68%, Protein: 20%, Net Carbs: 12%, Fiber: 25g

Shopping List for Week 3

Proteins

Beef, boneless sirloin steak, 12 ounces
Beef, 4 boneless sirloin mini-steaks (3 ounces each)
Chicken, pre-cooked, 2 breasts (about 1 pound)
Turkey, lean ground, 1½ pounds
Shrimp, any size, 1 pound
Eggs, 2 medium, 2 large
Cottage cheese, full-fat, 1 (4-ounce) container
Yogurt, plain full-fat Greek, 1 (5.3-ounce) container
Tuna, 1 (2-ounce) can, packed in water

Vegetables

Asparagus, 1½ pounds
Broccoli, 1 large crown (for about 4 cups florets)
Cabbage, pre-shredded, 1 (12-ounce) package (about 2 cups)
Carrots, 5 medium
Cauliflower rice, 1 (1-pound) package (2 cups)
Celery, 1 or 2 stalks
Cucumbers, 4 large, 1 small
Garlic, 6 cloves
Mushrooms, portobello or button, 1 pound (about 2 cups)
Onion, 1 medium white or yellow

Radishes, 8
Red bell peppers, 4
Spinach, 1 (10-ounce) package (about $3^1/_2$ cups)
Spinach, baby, 1 (16-ounce) package (about 4 cups)
Tomato, 1 ripe round
Mixed salad greens, 1 (10-ounce) package (about 3 cups)
Chickpeas, 1 (15-ounce) can

Fresh Herbs
Basil
Cilantro
Dill
Thyme

Fruits
Apple, 1 small
Avocados, 2 medium
Blackberries, $^1/_2$ pint
Blueberries, $^1/_2$ pint
Lemons, 2 to 3 medium
Raspberries, $^1/_2$ pint
Strawberries, 1 pint

Miscellaneous
Blue cheese, pre-crumbled, small package ($1^1/_2$ ounces)
Cheddar cheese, pre-shredded, large package (24 ounces)
Parmesan cheese, pre-grated, small package (about $^1/_4$ cup)
Milk, whole, 1 pint
Heavy cream, $^1/_2$ pint
Sour cream, 1 (8-ounce) container
Olives, 1 pound (2 cups)

Week 4

DAY 1

MEAL 1: PUMPKIN PANCAKES (PAGE 177)

Snack 1: Cucumber, Tomato, and Feta Salad (page 213)

MEAL 2: SPAGHETTI SQUASH WITH TURKEY, BACON, SPINACH, AND GOAT CHEESE (PAGE 197)

Snack 2: Turkey Mayo Lettuce Wraps (page 213)

Macros: Fat: 66%, Protein: 22%, Net Carbs: 12%, Fiber: 25g

DAY 2

MEAL 1: SPAGHETTI SQUASH WITH TURKEY, BACON, SPINACH, AND GOAT CHEESE (FROM DAY 1)

Snack 1: Deviled Eggs (page 214)

MEAL 2: BLT SALMON BURGERS (PAGE 192)

Snack 2: Crunchy Kale Chips with Pecans (page 210)

Macros: Fat: 67%, Protein: 25%, Net Carbs: 8%, Fiber: 28g

DAY 3

MEAL 1: PUMPKIN PANCAKES (FROM DAY 1)

Snack 1: Turkey Mayo Lettuce Wraps (from day 1)

MEAL 2: SPAGHETTI SQUASH WITH TURKEY, BACON, SPINACH, AND GOAT CHEESE (FROM DAY 1)

Snack 2: Strawberries with Chia Cream (page 217)

Macros: Fat: 67%, Protein: 21%, Net Carbs: 12%, Fiber: 27g

DAY 4

MEAL 1: PUMPKIN PANCAKES (FROM DAY 1)

Snack 1: Cheese and Walnuts (page 209)

MEAL 2: LEMON CHICKEN WITH CAPERS (PAGE 195)

Snack 2: 1/4 cup fresh blueberries

Macros: Fat: 69%, Protein: 21%, Net Carbs: 10%, Fiber: 25g

DAY 5

MEAL 1: SPAGHETTI SQUASH WITH TURKEY, BACON, SPINACH, AND GOAT CHEESE (FROM DAY 1)

Snack 1: Raspberry Almond Smoothie (page 219)

MEAL 2: PUMPKIN AND CHICKEN CURRY WITH CAULIFLOWER RICE (PAGE 186)

Snack 2: Creamy Avocado Dip (page 211) with veggie sticks

Macros: Fat: 67%, Protein: 20%, Net Carbs: 13%, Fiber: 30g

DAY 6

MEAL 1: PUMPKIN AND CHICKEN CURRY WITH CAULIFLOWER RICE (FROM DAY 5)

Snack 1: Peanut Butter Cup Smoothie (page 219)

MEAL 2: LEMON CHICKEN WITH CAPERS (PAGE 195) AND STEAMED BROCCOLI DRESSED WITH 1 TABLESPOON OLIVE OIL AND 1 TABLESPOON GROUND FLAXSEED

Snack 2: Pumpkin-Spiced Walnuts (page 208)

Macros: Fat: 66%, Protein: 22%, Net Carbs: 13%, Fiber: 27g

DAY 7

MEAL 1: CHOCOLATE STRAWBERRY SMOOTHIE (PAGE 173)

Snack 1: Creamy Avocado Dip (page 211) with 10 green beans

MEAL 2: EGG AND VEGETABLE SALAD (PAGE 188)

Snack 2: Naked Turkey Roll-Ups (page 214)

Macros: Fat: 69%, Protein: 20%, Net Carbs: 11%, Fiber: 31g

Shopping List for Week 4

Proteins

Bacon, uncured, 6 slices
Chicken, 1 (4-ounce) boneless, skinless breast
Chicken, pre-cooked breasts, 1 pound
Eggs, 6 large
Turkey, lean ground, 1 pound
Turkey, deli slices, about 2 ounces
Turkey bacon, 12 slices
Salmon, 1 (8-ounce) fillet
Yogurt, plain full-fat Greek, 1 (5.3-ounce) container

Vegetables

Broccoli, 1 crown (for about 4 cups florets)
Cauliflower rice, 1 package (about 1 cup)
Cucumbers, 2 medium
Garlic cloves, 2
Green beans, 1/4 pound (10 individual beans)
Green bell pepper, 1
Kale, 1 large bunch
Lettuce, butter or other, 1 small head
Onion, 1 medium red
Red bell pepper, 1
Spaghetti squash, 2 medium
Spinach, baby, 1 (16-ounce) package (about 4 cups)
Tomatoes, 2 ripe round
Tomatoes, cherry, 1 pint
Pumpkin puree, 1 (15-ounce) can (about 2 cups)

Fresh Herbs

Chives

Cilantro

Basil

Thai basil

Fruits

Avocados, 3 medium

Lemons, 2 medium

Raspberries, $^1/_2$ pint

Strawberries, 1 pint

Miscellaneous

Cheese sticks, small package

Cheddar cheese, pre-shredded, small package (about 1 cup)

Feta cheese, pre-crumbled, small package (about 1 ounce)

Goat cheese, 1 (4-ounce) package

Swiss cheese, 1 (2-ounce) piece

Heavy cream, $^1/_2$ pint

Sour cream, 1 (8-ounce) container

Olives, assorted, 8 ounces (about $^1/_4$ cup)

The Vegetarian Menus: Week 1

DAY 1

MEAL 1: FLAXSEED PANCAKES (PAGE 176)

Snack 1: Vegan Snack Bar (page 226)

MEAL 2: TOFU IN PEANUT SAUCE (PAGE 187)

Snack 2: Vegan Yogurt Parfait (page 223) with 2 tablespoons unsweetened coconut flakes

Macros: Fat: 66%, Protein: 18%, Net Carbs: 16%, Fiber: 33g

DAY 2

MEAL 1: TOFU IN PEANUT SAUCE (FROM DAY 1)

Snack 1: Cheesy Nuts (page 209)

MEAL 2: BBQ TEMPEH, GREENS, AND CAULIFLOWER RICE (PAGE 202)

Snack 2: Vegan Snack Bar (from day 1)

Macros: Fat: 71%, Protein: 19%, Net Carbs: 10%, Fiber: 31g

DAY 3

MEAL 1: FLAXSEED PANCAKES (FROM DAY 1)

Snack 1: Peanut Butter and Chocolate Chia Pudding (page 222)

MEAL 2: SLOW COOKER MUSHROOM STROGANOFF WITH CREAMY GARLIC CAULIFLOWER RICE (PAGE 200)

Snack 2: Vegan Cinnamon Roll Smoothie (page 220)

Macros: Fat: 65%, Protein: 20%, Net Carbs: 15%, Fiber: 49g

DAY 4

MEAL 1: SLOW COOKER MUSHROOM STROGANOFF WITH CREAMY GARLIC CAULIFLOWER RICE (FROM DAY 3)

Snack 1: Flaxseed Pancakes (from day 1)

MEAL 2: TOFU IN PEANUT SAUCE (FROM DAY 1)

Snack 2: Chia Pudding (page 221)

Macros: Fat: 69%, Protein: 14%, Net Carbs: 17%, Fiber: 31g

DAY 5

MEAL 1: BBQ TEMPEH, GREENS, AND CAULIFLOWER RICE (FROM DAY 2)

Snack 1: Chia Pudding (from day 4)

MEAL 2: TOFU IN PEANUT SAUCE (FROM DAY 1)

Snack 2: Chocolate Mocha Almonds with String Cheese (page 218)

Macros: Fat: 67%, Protein: 18%, Net Carbs: 15%, Fiber: 28g

DAY 6

MEAL 1: FLAXSEED PANCAKES (FROM DAY 1)

Snack 1: Peanut Butter and Chocolate Chia Pudding (from day 3)

MEAL 2: BBQ TEMPEH, GREENS, AND CAULIFLOWER RICE (FROM DAY 2)

Snack 2: Vegan Snack Bar (from day 1)

Macros: Fat: 67%, Protein: 17%, Net Carbs: 16%, Fiber: 43g

DAY 7

MEAL 1: BBQ TEMPEH, GREENS, AND CAULIFLOWER RICE (FROM DAY 2)

Snack 1: Vegan Snack Bar (from day 1)

MEAL 2: SLOW COOKER MUSHROOM STROGANOFF WITH CREAMY GARLIC CAULIFLOWER RICE (FROM DAY 3)

Snack 2: Vegan Yogurt Parfait (page 223)

Macros: Fat: 71%, Protein: 16%, Net Carbs: 13%, Fiber: 25g

Shopping List for Vegetarian Week 1

Proteins

Eggs, 4 large
Tempeh, 1 (1-pound) package
Tofu, firm, 1 (14-ounce) package (for about 1 3/8 cups)
Yogurt, plain full-fat Greek, 1 (5.3-ounce) container
Yogurt, plain unsweetened almond milk, 1 (5.3-ounce) container

Vegetables

Broccolini, 12 ounces (about 2 1/4 cups)
Cauliflower, 1 small head
Garlic cloves, 9
Kale, chopped, 1 (1-pound) package (about 6 cups)
Mushrooms, button, 2 (10-ounce) packages (about 5 cups)
Onion, 2 medium yellow

Fresh Herbs

Flat-leaf parsley
Ginger

Fruits

Blueberries, $^1/_2$ pint

Lemons, 2 medium

Miscellaneous

Blueberries, frozen, 1 (10-ounce) package (2 cups)

Cheese round, Babybel, 1

Orange juice, 4 ounces

Parmesan cheese, pre-grated, small package (about $^1/_2$ cup)

Protein powder, vanilla, 1 jar (such as KOS Organic Plant)

Vegetable broth, canned or jarred, 1 (15-ounce) container (about 2 cups)

Vegetarian Week 2

DAY 1

MEAL 1: BREAKFAST SALAD (PAGE 178)

Snack 1: Pear Slices and Ricotta Cheese (page 217)

MEAL 2: BLACKENED TOFU WITH SESAME BROCCOLI SLAW (PAGE 201)

Snack 2: 1 serving of Herbed White Bean Dip (page 212) with $^1/_2$ cup sugar snap peas, $^1/_2$ cup sliced radishes, 1 cup broccoli florets, 1 cup cauliflower florets

Macros: Fat: 68%, Protein: 16%, Net Carbs: 16%, Fiber: 27g

DAY 2

MEAL 1: GRAPE TOMATO AND PEA SALAD ON RICOTTA SPREAD (PAGE 180) WITH 1 TABLESPOON GROUND FLAXSEED

Snack 1: Hard-Boiled Egg with Avocado (page 214)

MEAL 2: BLACKENED TOFU WITH SESAME BROCCOLI SLAW (FROM DAY 1)

Snack 2: Peanut Butter–Mocha Smoothie (page 220)

Macros: Fat: 74%, Protein: 14%, Net Carbs: 12%, Fiber: 30g

DAY 3

MEAL 1: BLACKENED TOFU WITH SESAME BROCCOLI SLAW (FROM DAY 1)

Snack 1: 1 serving of Herbed White Bean Dip (from day 1) with $^1/_2$ cup sugar snap peas, $^1/_2$ cup sliced radishes, 1 cup broccoli florets, 1 cup cauliflower florets

MEAL 2: SPICY EDAMAME BOWL WITH CREAMY CHILI SAUCE (PAGE 206)

Snack 2: Green Almond Butter Smoothie (page 220)

Macros: Fat: 63%, Protein: 20%, Net Carbs: 17%, Fiber: 35g

DAY 4

MEAL 1: BREAKFAST SALAD (FROM DAY 1)

Snack 1: Blackened Tofu with Sesame Broccoli Slaw (from day 1)

MEAL 2: SPICY EDAMAME BOWL WITH CREAMY CHILI SAUCE (FROM DAY 3)

Snack 2: Chocolate Banana "Nice" Cream (page 226)

Macros: Fat: 71%, Protein: 15%, Net Carbs: 14%, Fiber: 32g

DAY 5

MEAL 1: SPICY EDAMAME BOWL WITH CREAMY CHILI SAUCE (FROM DAY 3)

Snack 1: Grape Tomato and Pea Salad on Ricotta Spread (from day 2)

MEAL 2: VEGGIE CHEESE ENCHILADAS WITH GRAIN-FREE TORTILLAS (PAGE 204)

Snack 2: Edamame Mash Salad (page 215)

Macros: Fat: 72%, Protein: 15%, Net Carbs: 13%, Fiber: 25g

DAY 6

MEAL 1: VEGAN PROTEIN SALAD (PAGE 181)

Snack 1: Hard-Boiled Egg with Avocado (page 214)

MEAL 2: SPICY EDAMAME BOWL WITH CREAMY CHILI SAUCE (FROM DAY 3)

Snack 2: ½ cup halved fresh strawberries and 5.3-ounce container of plain Greek-style almond milk yogurt

Macros: Fat: 67%, Protein: 18%, Net Carbs: 15%, Fiber: 30g

DAY 7

MEAL 1: VEGGIE CHEESE ENCHILADAS WITH GRAIN-FREE TORTILLAS (FROM DAY 5)

Snack 1: Edamame Mash Salad (from day 5)

MEAL 2: VEGAN PROTEIN SALAD (FROM DAY 6)

Snack 2: Chocolate Banana "Nice" Cream (from day 4)

Macros: Fat: 65%, Protein: 17%, Net Carbs: 19%, Fiber: 38g

Shopping List for Vegetarian Week 2

Proteins

Eggs, 10

Tempeh, 1 (16-ounce) package

Tofu, medium or firm, 1 (10-ounce) package

Tofu, extra firm, 1 (12-ounce) package

Yogurt, plain full-fat Greek, 1 (5.3-ounce) container

Yogurt, plain unsweetened almond milk, Greek style, 1 (5.3 ounce) container

Vegetables

Arugula, 1 ounce (about 1 cup)

Bell pepper, any type, 1

Broccoli slaw, 1 (14-ounce) bag

Coleslaw mix, 1 (14-ounce) bag

Garlic cloves, 7

Lettuce, romaine, 1 head

Onion, 1 medium red

Onion, 1 to 2 medium white or yellow

Red cabbage, pre-shredded, small package (about 1 cup)

Scallions, 6

Spinach, chopped, 1 (10-ounce) package (about 6 cups)

Spinach, baby, 1 small package (about 1 cup)

Tomatoes, cherry, 1 pint

Tomatoes, grape, 1 pint

Zucchini, 1 medium

Assorted vegetables: sugar snap peas, radishes, broccoli florets, cauliflower florets

Fresh Herbs

Cilantro

Dill

Ginger

Mint

Fruits

Avocados, 4 medium

Bananas, 2 ripe

Blueberries, $^1/_2$ pint

Lemons, 2 medium

Limes, 2 medium

Pear, 1 firm

Strawberries, 1 pint

Miscellaneous

Cacao nibs, small package (about 3 tablespoons)

Cheddar cheese, pre-shredded, 1 large package (about $1^1/_2$ cups)

Cannellini beans, 1 (15-ounce) can (about $^1/_2$ cup)

Edamame, frozen, 1 (10-ounce) package

Ricotta, 1 (15-ounce) container (about $1^1/_2$ cups)

Tomato sauce, no sugar added, 1 (15-ounce) can or jar (about $1^1/_2$ cups)

Vegetable broth, 1 (8-ounce) can or package (about 1 cup)

If You Want to DIY Your Meals

Don't want to follow the meal plans exactly? No problem; it's easy to create your own menus. The following are some examples.

Meal 1

Lunch salad. For meal 1, normally right around noon, it's a good idea to have a big mixed green salad with a quality protein like salmon, chicken, or eggs. If you're a vegan or vegetarian, top that salad with garbanzo beans or another legume. Sprinkle some nuts or seeds on top, and scatter on some avocado slices. Drizzle the salad with the juice of a lemon or some vinegar mixed with olive oil or avocado oil and herbs. A salad is such an easy vehicle for supplying your 70 percent of healthy fats like olive oil, avocado, nuts, and seeds at lunch.

Lettuce wrap. Prepare a lettuce wrap filled with tuna or egg salad, or hummus and veggies. A tomato stuffed with these foods is great, too. Meal 1 can even be a brunch with scrambled eggs, uncured, nitrate-free bacon, and sauteed veggies. Your main goal is proper fuel and a balance of it, including plenty of healthy fat!

For your beverage, at meals and snacks, have some more water, herbal tea, or coffee. (Watch caffeine, though, because it can worsen hot flashes.)

Meal 2

Protein + veg + starch. Pick a protein, a non-starchy vegetable, and maybe even a starchy vegetable like a sweet potato for a rounded meal. Good non-starchy vegetables are asparagus, broccoli, Brussels sprouts, cauliflower, and cauliflower rice. For starchy vegetables, choose sweet potatoes, winter squash, and potatoes.

Stir-fry + salad + potato. Try a stir-fry made with chicken tenders and vegetables served over cauliflower rice. To add more fat to the mix, cook the stir-fry in a high-quality fat like avocado oil. To keep it really simple, use 4 ounces of a lean steak (or other protein choice), a side salad with vinaigrette dressing, and a small baked potato topped with butter and sour cream.

Vegetarian meal. If you're looking for a vegetarian option, sauté some zucchini noodles with pesto or just olive oil and herbs, and top with grated Parmesan cheese.

In Summary

The meals all rely on proteins, veggies, salads, and fats in combination to provide just the right balance of nutrients that will control your hormones and metabolism.

Remember, you can enjoy two snacks a day in this program. Choose snacks that are whole, unprocessed foods whenever possible. In addition to nuts, consider cheese sticks, yogurt, olives, dill pickles, raw veggies, hard-boiled eggs, fresh berries, or uncured beef jerky to keep any hunger in check between meals.

You've probably noticed that all these meals are constructed of lots of healthy fats, a moderate amount of quality protein, generous servings of non-starchy carbs, and some starchy carbs. As I have explained, these foods play a crucial role in supporting weight loss, keeping inflammation at a low level, improving metabolism, supporting hormonal function, and enhancing overall health.

You may also have noticed that I didn't say anything about calorie counts or portion sizes. The Galveston Diet was designed so that you don't have to worry or obsess about those details. Because fats, proteins, and fiber-rich carbs make up most of the meals, you'll feel satisfied throughout the day and won't want to reach for that ol' sugary stuff or refined carbohydrates.

And by the time you're well into the program, you will intuitively know which foods to select to build your meals and you will eat properly and feel at your best. And don't forget to track your macros; that will help you be even more successful!

CHAPTER 9

The Galveston Diet Recipes

Since starting the Galveston Diet as an online program, I've been working with coaches, nutritionists, and chefs to develop more delicious, can't-wait-to-eat-this-again recipes that will keep you happy and on track. I love to cook and experiment with flavors and foods at home, so I've contributed some recipes as well.

In creating these recipes, we focused not only on flavor but also on ease of preparation. Let's face it—we're all busy. We need recipes that not only taste delicious but also can be made quickly.

These recipes are brand-new and not available online. They have been designed for the conventional Galveston Diet—which includes animal foods—but also for the vegan/vegetarian program, if you're someone who prefers to avoid animal products.

Enjoy!

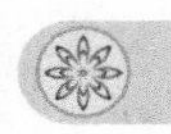

Mary Claire's Parfait or Smoothie

MAKES 1 SERVING

- $^3/_4$ cup plain full-fat Greek yogurt (such as Fage)
- $^1/_4$ cup sliced fresh strawberries
- $^1/_4$ cup fresh blueberries
- $^1/_4$ cup chopped walnuts
- 1 tablespoon ground flaxseed
- 1 tablespoon chia seeds
- 1 tablespoon hemp hearts
- 1 tablespoon unsweetened coconut flakes
- 2 to 3 ice cubes (for smoothie)
- Water, as needed (for smoothie)

AS A PARFAIT

Combine all the ingredients in a bowl and stir well. Serve at once.

AS A SMOOTHIE

Place all the ingredients except the water in a blender. Blend until smooth, adding a little water as necessary to reach the desired consistency.

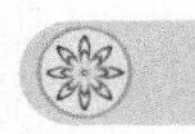

Chocolate Strawberry Smoothie

MAKES 1 SERVING

- 1 scoop protein powder
- 1 cup chopped fresh kale
- $^1/_2$ cup sliced fresh strawberries
- 1 tablespoon ground flaxseed
- 1 tablespoon unsweetened almond butter
- 1 tablespoon unsweetened cocoa powder
- $^1/_2$ cup coconut milk
- 2 tablespoons chia seeds
- Ice cubes (optional)

Place all the ingredients in a blender and blend until smooth.

Note: This can be made vegetarian or vegan, depending on the protein powder used.

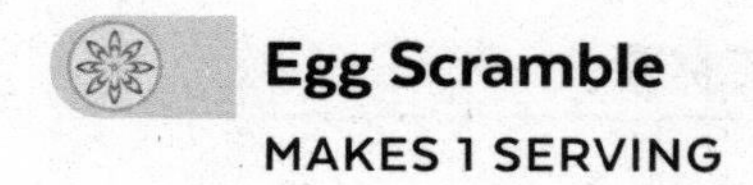

Egg Scramble

MAKES 1 SERVING

2 large eggs
Salt and black pepper
1 tablespoon butter
1 cup fresh spinach leaves
1/2 cup chopped fresh tomatoes
1 cup fresh raspberries (optional)

1. Crack the eggs into a medium bowl. Add a pinch of salt and pepper, and whisk until blended.
2. Melt the butter in a medium skillet over low heat.
3. Pour in the egg and cook until the edges of the eggs firm up. Gently fold the eggs over, then cook for another half-minute, pushing and folding them around the pan for another minute.
4. Add the spinach and tomatoes, and stir to incorporate. Continue pushing and folding the eggs until barely set. They should look a bit runny on top.
5. Serve the scrambled eggs with a small bowl of fresh raspberries, if desired.

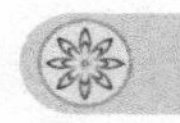

Cottage Cheese Omelet

MAKES 1 SERVING

2 large eggs
1 tablespoon milk
Salt and black pepper
1 tablespoon olive oil
1/2 cup spinach
3 tablespoons full-fat cottage cheese

1. In a medium bowl, combine the eggs, milk, and salt and pepper to taste, then whisk for 30 seconds.
2. Place the olive oil in a medium skillet over medium heat. When oil is shimmering, add the eggs and cook for 1 to 2 minutes, until mostly set.
3. Flip the omelet and spoon the spinach and cottage cheese onto one half of the omelet. Cook for another 1 to 2 minutes, then fold the omelet over the cottage cheese and serve.

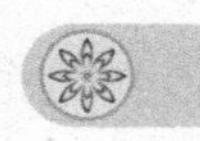

Poached Eggs with Cabbage Hash Browns

MAKES 1 SERVING

1 teaspoon olive oil
2 cups shredded green cabbage
$^1/_2$ cup sliced onion
2 medium eggs
Salt and black pepper
Dash of smoked paprika (optional)

1. Pour the olive oil into a medium skillet over medium heat. When the oil is shimmering, add the cabbage and onion and cook, stirring, until lightly browned, 8 to 10 minutes. The cabbage will shrink in size; just keep stirring it.
2. Transfer the sautéed cabbage and onion to a serving plate. Cover the dish and keep warm while you poach the eggs.
3. Fill a wide, medium pan with water and bring to a simmer over medium-low heat. When the water is at a bare simmer, break each egg into the water. After about 1 minute, turn the eggs over with a slotted spoon and simmer for an additional 3 to 4 minutes, or until the whites are firm.
4. Using the slotted spoon, transfer the eggs to the plate with the cabbage and onion. Season to taste with the salt and pepper, and add the smoked paprika, if using. Serve at once.

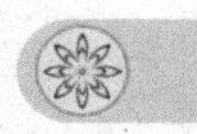

Avocado "For Life" Toast

MAKES 1 SERVING

1 tablespoon olive oil
2 large eggs
2 slices sprouted-grain bread (such as Food For Life brand)
1 avocado, halved, pitted, and sliced
Salt and black pepper
Red pepper flakes (optional)

1. Heat the olive oil over medium-high heat in a large skillet until shimmering. Add the eggs and cook to your preferred style, either fried or scrambled, about 3 minutes.
2. Meanwhile, toast the bread to desired doneness.
3. Place the toast on a serving plate. Add the avocado slices, then add the egg and season to taste with salt and pepper. Sprinkle with the red pepper flakes, if using. Serve at once.

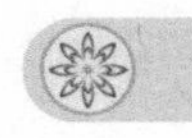

Flaxseed Pancakes

MAKES 4 SERVINGS

1 cup ground flaxseed

4 large eggs, lightly beaten

$^1/_3$ cup unsweetened almond milk (or other milk), or more as needed

2 teaspoons fresh lemon juice

1 teaspoon baking soda

1 teaspoon vanilla extract

1 teaspoon ground cinnamon

$^1/_8$ teaspoon salt

$^1/_2$ tablespoon coconut oil

4 tablespoons unsweetened almond butter

2 cups frozen blueberries

1. In a large bowl, combine the flaxseed, eggs, almond milk, lemon juice, baking soda, vanilla, cinnamon, and salt. If the mixture is too thick, add more almond milk or water to achieve a batter consistency.
2. Heat a large skillet over medium heat and add the coconut oil. When melted and hot, pour about $^1/_4$ cup of the batter for each of 2 or 3 pancakes and gently spread it with a spoon. Let cook on one side for 2 to 3 minutes, or until the edges begin to firm and bubbles appear, then flip and cook on the opposite side for another 2 to 3 minutes. Keep the cooked pancakes warm on a covered plate while you make any more pancakes with the remaining batter.
3. Meanwhile, melt the almond butter in a small bowl in the microwave. Place the frozen blueberries in a medium bowl and microwave until they are no longer frozen, have warmed slightly, and become juicy.
4. Place the pancakes on serving plates, drizzle with the melted almond butter, and sprinkle with the blueberries.

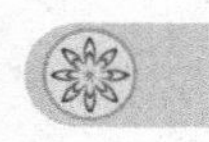

Pumpkin Pancakes

MAKES 3 SERVINGS

2 tablespoons ground flaxseed

$^{3}/_{4}$ cup almond flour

1 tablespoon coconut flour

1 teaspoon stevia

$^{1}/_{2}$ teaspoon baking powder

$^{1}/_{2}$ teaspoon pumpkin pie spice

$^{1}/_{2}$ cup canned pumpkin puree

2 large eggs, lightly beaten

1 tablespoon avocado oil

6 tablespoons unsweetened almond butter

3 tablespoons pumpkin seeds

1. In a large bowl, combine the flaxseed, flours, stevia, baking powder, and pumpkin pie spice. Add the pumpkin and the eggs. Stir well to blend and moisten all the ingredients.
2. Heat a large skillet or griddle over medium heat. When hot, add $^{1}/_{2}$ tablespoon of the avocado oil to coat the pan, then add 2 or 3 large spoonfuls of the batter. The batter should spread to make pancakes 3 to 4 inches in diameter.
3. Cook the pancakes on the first side for about 3 minutes, then flip and cook on the other side for an additional 2 to 3 minutes. When lightly browned, transfer to a plate, cover, and keep warm. Add the remaining $^{1}/_{2}$ tablespoon avocado oil to the pan and then additional spoonfuls of the batter. Cook as for the first batch.
4. Transfer the pancakes to serving plates, top with the almond butter and pumpkin seeds, and serve.

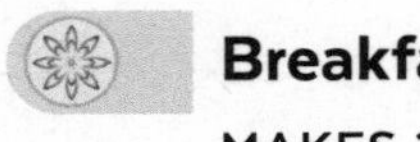

Breakfast Salad

MAKES 2 SERVINGS

3 tablespoons avocado oil mayonnaise

1 garlic clove, crushed

2 teaspoons fresh lemon juice

4 cups torn romaine lettuce leaves

1 cup halved cherry tomatoes

1 medium avocado, halved, pitted, and sliced

1/4 small onion, sliced

Salt and black pepper

1/2 cup pumpkin seeds

4 large eggs, hard-boiled, peeled, and quartered

1. In a small bowl, blend the mayonnaise, garlic, and lemon juice to make the dressing.
2. Arrange the lettuce on 2 serving plates. To each plate, add some of the cherry tomatoes, avocado, and onion. Season to taste with salt and pepper. Top with the pumpkin seeds and egg quarters, then drizzle with the dressing and serve.

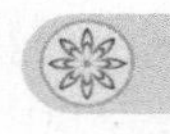

Chicken and BLT Wrap

MAKES 2 SERVINGS

2 large bibb or romaine lettuce leaves

1 avocado, halved, pitted, and sliced

1 cup (6 ounces) shredded rotisserie-cooked chicken breast

1/2 cup chopped fresh tomato

2 slices turkey bacon

4 tablespoons ranch dressing (homemade or brand such as Primal Kitchen)

1/8 teaspoon black pepper

1/4 cup (1 ounce) grated cheddar cheese

1. Place the lettuce leaves on a board and flatten slightly. To each leaf add some of the avocado and then the chicken, tomato, and turkey bacon. Drizzle with the dressing, season with the pepper, and sprinkle on the cheese.
2. Fold up the sides of the leaf and serve at once.

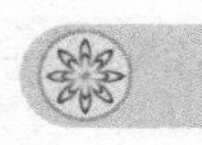

Tuna Salad with Snacky Side Salad

MAKES 1 SERVING

FOR THE TUNA SALAD

1 (2-ounce) can tuna packed in water, drained

1 tablespoon chopped red onion

2 tablespoons avocado oil mayonnaise

2 tablespoons chopped pecans

FOR THE SIDE SALAD

1 cup mixed salad greens

$^{1}/_{2}$ cup chopped ripe tomato

1 medium carrot, chopped

1 celery stalk, chopped

1 tablespoon olive oil

1 lemon, juiced

1. Make the tuna salad: Empty the can of tuna into a medium bowl and add the onion, mayonnaise, and pecans. Stir to blend well.
2. Make the side salad: Place the salad greens, tomato, carrot, and celery in a medium salad bowl. Drizzle on the olive oil and lemon juice, then gently toss.
3. Assemble the salad: Top the greens with the tuna salad and serve.

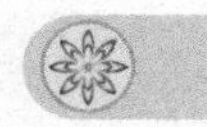

TGD Cobb Salad

MAKES 4 SERVINGS

8 cups chopped romaine lettuce

2 cups (12 ounces) shredded rotisserie-cooked chicken breast

12 slices turkey bacon

2 avocados, halved, pitted, and chopped

8 hard-boiled eggs

1 $^{1}/_{2}$ cups cherry tomatoes, halved

$^{1}/_{2}$ cup ranch dressing (homemade or brand such as Primal Kitchen)

4 tablespoons sunflower seeds

In a large bowl, combine the lettuce with the chicken, turkey bacon, avocado, eggs, and tomatoes. Spoon on the dressing and toss well. Sprinkle with the sunflower seeds and serve.

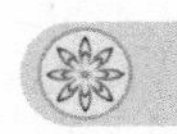

Grape Tomato and Pea Salad on Ricotta Spread

MAKES 1 SERVING

FOR THE SALAD

1 cup full-fat ricotta

1 tablespoon olive oil

$^1/_2$ teaspoon salt

1 cup baby arugula

1 cup baby spinach

$^1/_2$ cup stemmed and halved sugar snap peas

$^1/_2$ cup grape tomatoes, halved

FOR THE DRESSING

2 tablespoons white balsamic vinegar

1 cup chopped fresh basil

2 tablespoons olive oil

Pinch of red pepper flakes

Salt and black pepper

1. Prepare the salad: Place the ricotta, olive oil, and salt in a food processor and process until creamy. Transfer the spread to a serving plate.
2. In a large bowl, toss together the arugula, spinach, sugar snap peas, and grape tomatoes.
3. Make the dressing: In a blender or food processor, combine the dressing ingredients until emulsified.
4. Assemble: Pour the dressing over the greens and mix thoroughly, then place atop the ricotta spread on the plate. Serve.

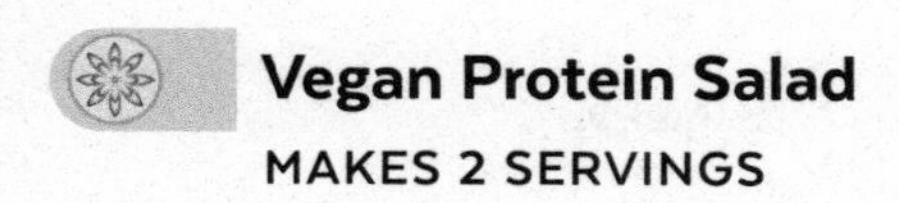

Vegan Protein Salad

MAKES 2 SERVINGS

FOR THE MARINATED TEMPEH

2 tablespoons balsamic vinegar

1 tablespoon tamari or soy sauce

1 tablespoon pure maple syrup

1/2 teaspoon garlic powder

Pinch of salt and black pepper

1/2 block (about 4 ounces) tempeh, cut into cubes

FOR THE BAKED TOFU

1/2 block (about 5 ounces) medium or firm tofu, cut into cubes

1/2 teaspoon garlic powder

1 tablespoon tamari or soy sauce

Pinch of salt and black pepper

FOR THE SALAD

1 cup chopped and steamed broccoli

2 cups lightly chopped fresh arugula

1 cup diced cucumber

1 avocado, halved, pitted, and chopped

4 tablespoons hemp seeds

1 tablespoon tahini

1 tablespoon olive oil

Fresh lemon juice

1. Make the tempeh: Mix the balsamic vinegar, tamari, maple syrup, garlic powder, and salt and pepper in a shallow dish. Add the tempeh and let soak for at least 2 hours and up to overnight.
2. When ready, preheat the oven to 400°F. Either spray a small baking dish with nonstick cooking spray or line it with a silicone baking mat.
3. Transfer the tempeh cubes to the baking dish and bake the tempeh for 20 minutes. Toss the tempeh cubes with a bit of the leftover marinade, if desired. Keep the oven turned on.
4. Make the tofu: Toss the tofu cubes with the garlic powder, tamari, and salt and pepper and bake at 400°F for 30 minutes, until lightly browned. (If desired, bake it at the same time as you bake the tempeh.)
5. Assemble the salad: Place the broccoli, arugula, cucumber, and avocado in a large salad bowl. Add the baked tempeh and tofu cubes and mix well. Sprinkle on the hemp seeds. Drizzle on the tahini and olive oil, then toss to coat everything well with the dressing. Finish the salad with a spritz of fresh lemon juice and serve.

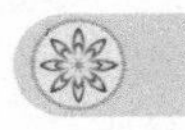

Roasted Tomato Bisque

MAKES 4 SERVINGS

4 tablespoons olive oil
8 medium Roma (plum) tomatoes
4 garlic cloves, minced
1 (15-ounce) can cannellini beans
2 cups chicken broth
Salt and black pepper
1 cup heavy cream
Fresh basil, julienned (optional)

1. Preheat the oven to 400°F. Lightly oil a baking sheet with the olive oil.
2. Halve the tomatoes and place tomatoes on the baking sheet and sprinkle with the garlic. Roast for 20 to 25 minutes, or until the tomatoes are soft.
3. Transfer the tomatoes and garlic to a blender and add the beans. Process until smooth.
4. Pour the tomato-bean puree into a medium pot set over medium heat. Add the broth, heat through, and then season to taste with the salt and pepper.
5. Stir in the cream and then ladle the soup into individual bowls. Sprinkle with the basil, if using, and serve.

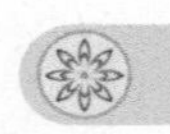

Chicken Taco Salad

MAKES 1 SERVING

3/4 cup chopped cooked chicken breast
Pinch each of chili powder, ground cumin, oregano, or other desired spices
1/2 teaspoon garlic salt
2 tablespoons Easy Guacamole (page 211)
2 tablespoons sour cream
2 tablespoons salsa fresca
1/2 cup canned black beans, rinsed and drained
2 cups mixed torn salad greens

Place the chicken in a large bowl and season with the spices and garlic salt. Add the guacamole, sour cream, salsa, and beans, and toss well. Place the salad greens on a dinner plate, top with the chicken/bean mixture, and serve.

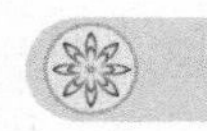

Tuna Salad over Mixed Greens

MAKES 1 SERVING

2 cups torn mixed salad greens

1 (3-ounce) can tuna packed in water, drained

1 tablespoon minced onion

2 tablespoons olive oil mayonnaise or avocado oil mayonnaise

2 tablespoons chopped pecans

1. Place the salad greens in a medium salad bowl.
2. Combine the tuna, onion, and mayonnaise in a small bowl, then spoon it over the greens and top with the pecans.

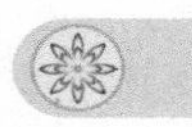

Sesame Ginger Pork with Green Beans

MAKES 4 SERVINGS

1/4 cup sesame seeds

Nonstick cooking spray

8 ounces boneless pork loin, cut into 1/2-inch strips

Salt and black pepper

2 tablespoons coconut oil

4 garlic cloves, minced

2 teaspoons grated fresh ginger

2 cups trimmed fresh green beans

2 teaspoons tamari

1 tablespoon toasted sesame oil

1. Place the sesame seeds in a small skillet over medium heat and toast until fragrant and lightly browned.
2. Lightly coat a medium skillet with the cooking spray, then add the pork strips and cook for 6 to 8 minutes, until lightly browned (or to 145°F). Season the pork to taste with the salt and pepper, then transfer to a plate.
3. Add the coconut oil to the skillet and heat for 45 seconds. Add the garlic, ginger, and green beans to the pan, and sauté for 6 to 8 minutes, until the beans are tender.
4. Add the pork strips back to the skillet and drizzle in the tamari. Toss the beans and pork until flavors are combined.
5. Transfer to individual plates, then sprinkle with the toasted sesame seeds and drizzle with the toasted sesame oil.

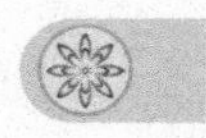

Bell Peppers Stuffed with Turkey and Cauliflower Rice

MAKES 4 SERVINGS

Nonstick cooking spray

4 tablespoons coconut oil

12 ounces lean ground turkey

1 cup cauliflower rice

2 garlic cloves, minced

Ground cumin

Paprika

Black pepper

Minced fresh cilantro

2 large red bell peppers, cored and sliced in half lengthwise

2 cups (8 ounces) shredded cheddar cheese

1. Preheat the oven to 300°F. Lightly coat a medium baking dish with the cooking spray.
2. Add the coconut oil to a medium skillet over medium heat. When the oil is melted and warm, add the turkey and cook for 5 to 8 minutes, until no longer pink.
3. Transfer the turkey to a large bowl and add the cauliflower rice and garlic. Season to taste with the cumin, paprika, pepper, and cilantro. Mix well.
4. Arrange the peppers on a board. Stuff the turkey mixture into the pepper halves, patting the mixture firmly into the pieces, then top the stuffed peppers with the cheese.
5. Place the stuffed peppers in the baking dish and bake for 10 minutes, or until the cheese is lightly browned on top.

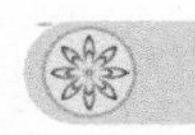

Shrimp and Asparagus

MAKES 4 SERVINGS

2 tablespoons butter

2 tablespoons olive oil

1 pound shrimp, peeled and deveined

1 pound fresh asparagus, coarse ends trimmed and remainder sliced

1 tablespoon minced garlic

Salt and black pepper

Dash of smoked paprika (optional)

$^1/_2$ fresh lemon, zested and juiced

$^1/_4$ cup (2 ounces) grated Parmesan cheese

2 tablespoons ground flaxseed

1. In a large skillet set over medium heat, melt the butter and add the olive oil. When oil is shimmering, add the shrimp and asparagus and lightly sauté for 3 to 4 minutes.
2. Add the garlic, stir well, then season with the salt and pepper. Sprinkle on the paprika, if using, then add the lemon zest and the lemon juice. Heat and stir, cooking until the shrimp is pink throughout and the asparagus is tender.
3. Meanwhile, in a small bowl, combine the cheese and flaxseed.
4. When ready to serve, sprinkle the cheese-flaxseed mixture over the shrimp and asparagus, stir to coat, then serve.

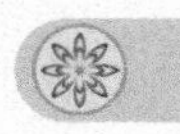

Pumpkin and Chicken Curry with Cauliflower Rice

MAKES 2 SERVINGS

2 tablespoons coconut oil

1 (4-ounce) skinless, boneless chicken breast or thigh, cubed

½ cup chopped red bell pepper

⅔ cup canned pumpkin puree

Curry powder

Other spices of choice

1 cup unsweetened coconut milk

Fresh Thai basil, julienned

1 cup cauliflower rice, cooked according to package instructions

1. In a medium skillet over medium heat, heat the coconut oil until melted and hot.
2. Add the chicken and cook for 3 to 4 minutes, stirring continuously, until almost cooked through.
3. Add the red pepper, pumpkin puree, curry powder, and spices of your choice. Stir well to coat the ingredients with the seasonings.
4. Add the coconut milk, increase the heat to medium-high, and bring to a boil. Reduce the heat to a simmer and cook slowly for 10 minutes.
5. Adjust the spices according to your taste, then transfer the curry to bowls and garnish with the Thai basil. Serve with the cauliflower rice.

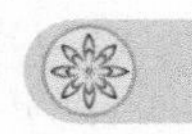

Tofu in Peanut Sauce

MAKES 4 SERVINGS

1 (14-ounce) square firm tofu

$^1/_4$ cup no-sugar-added peanut butter

2 tablespoons tamari

2 tablespoons water

3 tablespoons ground turmeric

1 teaspoon toasted sesame oil

$^1/_2$ teaspoon red pepper flakes

1 tablespoon grated fresh ginger

2 $^1/_4$ cups chopped fresh broccolini

1 tablespoon coconut oil

1. Sandwich the tofu between 2 paper towels and 2 plates. Place a heavy item like a can on the top plate, and press the tofu for at least 30 minutes. Then cut the tofu into $^1/_2$-inch cubes; you should have about 1 $^1/_2$ cups.
2. Combine the peanut butter, tamari, and water. Add the turmeric, sesame oil, red pepper flakes, and ginger.
3. Steam or boil the broccolini until tender, about 5 minutes. Keep warm.
4. Heat the coconut oil in a large skillet over medium heat and, when melted, add the tofu and cook for 10 to 15 minutes, occasionally turning, until lightly browned.
5. Stir in the sauce and blend well. Transfer to serving bowls and serve with the warm broccolini.

Note: You can also serve this over cauliflower rice.

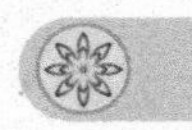

Egg and Vegetable Salad

MAKES 1 SERVING

2 hard-boiled large eggs, peeled and quartered

2 tablespoons olive oil mayonnaise or avocado oil mayonnaise

1 teaspoon spicy brown mustard

1 tablespoon apple cider vinegar

$^1/_4$ cup sliced pitted olives

1 small cucumber, chopped

1 tablespoon diced red onion

1 celery stalk, diced

1 medium carrot, diced

2 large butter, bibb, or other lettuce leaves

1. In a medium bowl, mash the eggs with the mayonnaise, mustard, and vinegar. Blend well. Stir in the olives.
2. In another bowl, combine the cucumber, onion, celery, and carrot.
3. Arrange the lettuce leaves on a serving plate. Spoon on the cucumber mix, then spoon the egg salad on top. Serve.

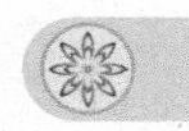

Grilled Chicken Salad

MAKES 4 SERVINGS

4 cups water

$^1/_4$ cup kosher salt

2 large boneless, skinless chicken breasts (about 1 pound), cut into 4 pieces

3 tablespoons olive oil, plus more for the grill

1 $^1/_2$ teaspoons paprika

1 head romaine lettuce, chopped

1 lemon, juiced

1. Combine the water and salt in a large bowl, stirring to dissolve the salt. Add the chicken to the bowl and refrigerate for 30 minutes. The brining adds moisture to the chicken.
2. If using an outdoor grill, preheat one side of the grill on high and the other side on medium. Alternatively, place a stovetop grill pan over medium-high heat.
3. Pat the chicken dry. Place in a medium bowl, add the olive oil and paprika, and swish it around to coat the breasts.
4. Brush the grill grates with a little olive oil, then place the chicken on the hot side of the grill (or in the grill pan). Grill, without disturbing, until the chicken pieces start getting some grill marks. (Peek underneath to check.) Turn the pieces over and move them to the cooler side of the grill (or reduce the heat to medium under the grill pan). Continue to grill the chicken until an instant-read thermometer inserted in the thickest part reaches 155°F.
5. Transfer the chicken to a platter and cover with foil. Let rest for about 10 minutes.
6. Arrange the romaine on a serving platter. Place the chicken atop the romaine and sprinkle with the lemon juice. Serve.

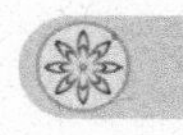

Portobello Pizzas

MAKES 2 SERVINGS

2 tablespoons olive oil

1/2 red onion, chopped

4 large portobello mushrooms, caps left whole and stems chopped

1/2 cup grape tomatoes, halved

Salt and black pepper

1/2 cup (about 2 ounces) shredded mozzarella cheese

1/4 cup (about 1 ounce) shredded Parmesan cheese

1/4 cup julienned fresh basil

1. Heat the olive oil in a large skillet over medium heat. Add the red onion and sauté 3 to 4 minutes, until lightly softened, then add the mushroom stems and the grape tomatoes, reduce the heat to medium-low, and simmer for 5 minutes, until the tomatoes are paste-like. Season to taste with the salt and pepper. Transfer the mixture to a small bowl.
2. Add the mushroom caps to the skillet and cook over medium heat for 3 to 4 minutes on each side.
3. Spread the tomato mixture in the mushroom caps, still in the skillet, and sprinkle on the cheeses. Lower the heat to medium-low, cover, and simmer until the cheeses melt, about 5 minutes.
4. Transfer the mushroom "pizzas" to serving plates. Top with the basil and serve.

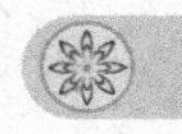

Cheeseburger Lettuce Sliders

MAKES 2 SERVINGS

6 ounces grass-fed 90% lean ground beef

Salt and black pepper

1 tablespoon olive oil

4 large bibb or romaine lettuce leaves

2 slices cheddar cheese

2 tablespoons olive oil mayonnaise

2 slices ripe tomato

1 avocado

2 small onion slices

2 slices dill pickle

1. Shape the beef into 4 equal patties. Season them with some salt and pepper.
2. Add the olive oil to a medium skillet over medium heat. When the oil is shimmering, add the patties and cook for 4 to 5 minutes on one side, then flip and continue to cook for another 4 minutes, or until they are medium-well.
3. Arrange 2 of the lettuce leaves on serving plates, then top with the patties, followed by the cheese, mayo, tomato, avocado, onion, and pickle. Add the remaining lettuce leaves to form a "bun." Serve.

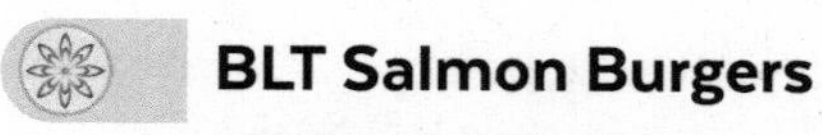

BLT Salmon Burgers

MAKES 4 SERVINGS

16 slices turkey bacon, cut in half crosswise

1 (8-ounce) salmon fillet, poached, skin removed, and cooled

2 to 3 tablespoons mayonnaise

Salt and black pepper

2 tablespoons olive oil

2 avocados, halved, pitted, and mashed

4 tablespoons ground flaxseed

Juice of $^1/_2$ lemon

3 tablespoons minced fresh chives

4 butter, bibb, or other lettuce leaves

2 ripe tomatoes, cut into 4 slices

1. Preheat the oven to 400°F. Line a rimmed baking sheet with aluminum foil, then place a baking rack into the baking sheet.
2. Make 4 bacon weaves. Cover a portion of your work space with parchment or wax paper. Arrange 3 bacon half-strips in a row on the parchment. Fold the middle piece back by two-thirds. Lay another half-strip of bacon across the 3 pieces at the fold. Unfold the piece over the newly added strip. Now fold the 2 side strips back by half and lay another half-strip over the rows at the new folds. Fold the side pieces back down and fold up the middle piece again by one-third. Finally, lay another bacon half-strip across the fold and tuck it underneath the end slices. Flatten the bacon weave with a rolling pin or the bottom of a skillet, then transfer to the oven rack on the baking sheet. Repeat, making 3 more bacon weaves.
3. Bake until the bacon is crisp, about 25 minutes. Drain the bacon weaves on a paper towel–lined plate. Cover to keep warm.
4. Make the salmon burgers: Mash the salmon in a medium bowl, with mayonnaise as needed to shape into 4 patties. Season with some salt and pepper.
5. Place a medium skillet over medium-high heat and add the olive oil. When the oil is shimmering, add the salmon patties and cook for about 8 minutes, flipping once, until lightly browned on both sides. Keep warm.
6. In a medium bowl, stir together the avocado, flaxseed, lemon juice, and chives.
7. Place a bacon weave on each of 4 serving plates, and spread with some of the avocado mixture. Add the salmon burger, a lettuce leaf, and a tomato slice. Serve.

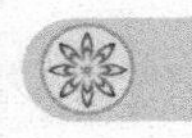

Baked Salmon with Grilled Summer Squash

MAKES 4 SERVINGS

FOR THE SQUASH

Oil for brushing the grill

1 medium yellow squash, sliced

1 medium zucchini, sliced

1 tablespoon unsalted butter, melted

1 lemon, zested and juiced

Salt and black pepper

1 teaspoon cayenne pepper, or to taste

FOR THE SALMON

Nonstick cooking spray

1 lemon, thinly sliced

1 large salmon fillet (about 3 pounds)

Salt and black pepper

6 tablespoons (3/4 stick) butter, melted

1 tablespoon honey

3 garlic cloves, minced

1 teaspoon chopped fresh thyme

1 teaspoon dried oregano

Sprigs of fresh parsley, for garnish

1. Grill the squash: Preheat an outdoor grill to medium and lightly oil the grill.
2. Place the yellow squash and zucchini slices on separate squares of aluminum foil. Pour the melted butter over the slices and sprinkle with the lemon zest and juice. Season with the salt, pepper, and cayenne. Fold up and wrap the squash in the aluminum foil. Place the squash packets on the preheated grill and grill until tender, about 30 minutes.
3. Bake the salmon: While the squash is grilling, preheat the oven to 350°F. Line a large-rimmed baking sheet with foil and spray with cooking spray.
4. Arrange the lemon slices in an even layer in the center of the baking sheet. Season both sides of the salmon with salt and pepper, and place on top of the lemon slices.
5. In a small bowl, whisk together the butter, honey, garlic, thyme, and oregano. Pour this mixture over the salmon and fold the foil up and around it.
6. Bake the salmon until it is cooked through and flakes easily, 15 to 20 minutes. Turn the oven on to broil, and broil the salmon for 2 minutes, or until the top is lightly browned and the butter mixture around it has thickened.
7. Remove the squash packets from the grill. Transfer the salmon to a serving platter. Garnish with the parsley sprigs, and unwrap and serve the grilled squash alongside.

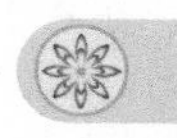

Grilled Shrimp with Broiled Tomato Bites

MAKES 4 SERVINGS

FOR THE SHRIMP

1/3 cup olive oil
2 tablespoons fresh lemon juice
1 teaspoon salt
1/4 teaspoon black pepper
1 teaspoon Italian seasoning
2 teaspoons minced garlic
1 pound large shrimp, peeled and deveined
4 bamboo skewers
Chopped fresh parsley, for garnish
Lemon wedges, for serving

FOR THE TOMATOES

Nonstick cooking spray
8 small ripe tomatoes
2 tablespoons olive oil
1/4 cup (1 ounce) grated Parmesan cheese

1. Marinate the shrimp: Place the olive oil, lemon juice, salt, pepper, Italian seasoning, and garlic in a large resealable plastic bag. Seal and shake to combine. Place the shrimp in a medium baking dish and spread them out. Pour the marinade from the bag over the shrimp. Place in the refrigerator to marinate for at least 15 minutes and up to 2 hours. Meanwhile, soak the skewers in water to moisten them.
2. Prepare the tomatoes: Set the oven rack for broiling. Coat a small, shallow baking dish with the cooking spray. Cut the tomatoes into halves, then cut a small sliver from the bottom of each so it can stand upright in the baking dish. Brush the olive oil on top of the tomatoes and sprinkle with the Parmesan.
3. Preheat the grill to medium hot. Preheat the broiler as well. Thread the shrimp onto the skewers. Place the skewers on the grill and cook for 2 to 3 minutes on each side, or until the shrimp are pink and opaque. Transfer the skewers to a serving platter and cover to keep warm.
4. Place the baking dish in the broiler and broil the tomatoes for 3 minutes, or until the cheese topping is lightly toasted. Watch carefully that the tomatoes do not burn.
5. Transfer the tomatoes to the platter with the skewers and arrange around them. Sprinkle the shrimp with the parsley and serve with the lemon wedges.

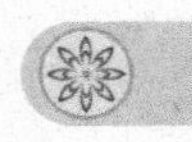

Lemon Chicken with Capers

MAKES 4 SERVINGS

4 skinless, boneless chicken breast halves (about 1 pound)

Salt and black pepper

4 tablespoons ghee (clarified butter) or olive oil

2 lemons, 1 juiced and 1 sliced

1 garlic clove, sliced

2 tablespoons drained capers

1 large onion, sliced

4 cups trimmed green beans

$^1/_4$ cup slivered almonds, toasted

1. Pat the chicken pieces dry and season to taste with salt and pepper.
2. In a large skillet over medium-high heat, add 1 tablespoon of the ghee and, when shimmering, add the chicken pieces. Cook, flipping once, for 8 to 10 minutes, until cooked through. Transfer the chicken to a plate. Cover and keep warm.
3. To the skillet, add the lemon juice, 1 tablespoon of the ghee, the garlic, and capers and bring to a simmer over medium-high heat. Add the lemon slices, then return the chicken to the skillet and reduce the heat. Simmer the chicken for 5 minutes.
4. In another medium skillet over medium heat, warm the remaining 2 tablespoons ghee. When shimmering, add the onion and beans, and cook until the onion is translucent and the beans are fork-tender, about 3 minutes.
5. Toss the slivered almonds into the beans and stir to combine.
6. Arrange the chicken on a serving platter and accompany with the onion and beans.

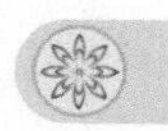

Broccoli and Cheese Chicken Bake

MAKES 4 SERVINGS

3 cups chopped or shredded cooked chicken breast

4 cups broccoli florets (fresh or frozen), cooked until fork-tender

2 tablespoons olive oil

½ cup sour cream

½ cup heavy cream

1 garlic clove, minced

1 teaspoon minced fresh basil

Salt and black pepper

1 cup (4 ounces) shredded cheddar cheese

1. Preheat the oven to 375°F.
2. Place the chicken in a large casserole dish, add the broccoli, and toss with olive oil.
3. In a medium bowl, combine the sour cream, heavy cream, garlic, and basil. Season to taste with the salt and pepper.
4. Pour the sauce into the casserole and stir to coat the chicken and broccoli. Sprinkle the top with the cheese and bake for 7 to 10 minutes, or until heated through and bubbly. Serve.

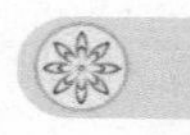

Sirloin, Spinach, and Blue Cheese Salad with Pecans

MAKES 4 SERVINGS

2 cups fresh spinach leaves

3 tablespoons crumbled blue cheese

2 tablespoons chopped pecans

2 tablespoons olive oil

Juice of ½ lemon

Salt and black pepper

1 (12-ounce) boneless sirloin steak, grilled or broiled as desired and thinly sliced

1. In a large salad bowl, toss the spinach, blue cheese, and pecans. Drizzle on the olive oil and lemon juice, and toss to coat everything well with the dressing. Season to taste with the salt and pepper.
2. Place the salad on individual plates, then add the steak slices. Serve.

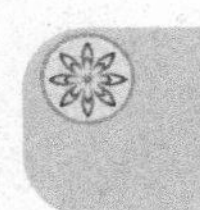

Spaghetti Squash with Turkey, Bacon, Spinach, and Goat Cheese

MAKES 4 SERVINGS

2 medium spaghetti squash

2 tablespoons olive oil

Salt and black pepper

6 slices bacon

1 pound lean ground turkey

1/4 cup dry white wine

4 cups baby spinach

1 (4-ounce) piece of goat cheese

1. Preheat the oven to 400°F. Line a rimmed baking sheet with aluminum foil.
2. Cut the stem ends off the squash. Stand the squash upright on their flat ends and cut in half lengthwise. Scoop out the seeds, then season the flesh with the olive oil and some salt and pepper.
3. Place the squash halves cut-side down on the baking sheet. Bake for 40 minutes to 1 hour, or until a fork inserted in the squash flesh goes in easily.
4. While the squash is cooking, using a large skillet set over medium heat, cook the bacon until crisp, about 10 minutes. Set the bacon aside to drain on a plate lined with paper towels. Add the turkey to the skillet and brown the meat, stirring well, for 5 to 8 minutes. Transfer the turkey to a large bowl and drain off most of the fat in the skillet, leaving about 1 tablespoon in the pan.
5. With the skillet over medium heat, pour in the wine and use a wooden spoon to scrape up the browned bits on the bottom. Cook and stir for about 1 minute to reduce the wine by about half.
6. Add the spinach to the skillet, stirring and heating until it wilts, about 3 minutes. Then crumble in the goat cheese and stir to soften and melt slightly for about 3 minutes.
7. Crumble the bacon and stir it into the turkey. Add the spinach-cheese mixture and stir to blend.
8. Remove the squash from the oven. When it's cool enough to handle, use a fork to comb out the flesh from the rinds of the squash, making "spaghetti" strands, and place in four serving bowls.
9. Top each squash mixture with the turkey, bacon, and spinach mixture and serve.

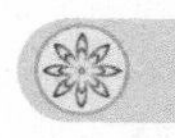

Meatloaf with Cauliflower Mash

MAKES 6 SERVINGS

2 tablespoons olive oil

$^{1}/_{4}$ cup chopped onion

1 $^{1}/_{2}$ pounds lean, grass-fed ground beef

1 cup almond flour

2 large eggs

$^{1}/_{3}$ cup no-sugar-added tomato sauce

$^{1}/_{2}$ cup (about 2 ounces) grated Parmesan cheese

$^{1}/_{2}$ teaspoon salt

$^{1}/_{2}$ teaspoon black pepper

$^{1}/_{2}$ teaspoon garlic powder

3 cups mashed cauliflower (from frozen or homemade), warmed

6 tablespoons ($^{3}/_{4}$ stick) butter (optional)

1. Preheat the oven to 350°F.
2. Heat the olive oil in a small skillet, add the onion, and sauté until it turns translucent, about 3 minutes.
3. In a large bowl, combine the ground beef, sautéed onion, almond flour, eggs, tomato sauce, cheese, salt, pepper, and garlic powder. Shape the mixture into a firm oval loaf.
4. Place the loaf in a shallow baking pan or loaf pan, and bake for 1 hour.
5. Carefully remove the loaf from the pan, discarding the surrounding fat, and transfer to a serving platter. Let rest for about 10 minutes, then slice for serving. Place the slices on plates and accompany with portions of the mashed cauliflower. If desired, top each serving of cauliflower with a generous pat of butter.

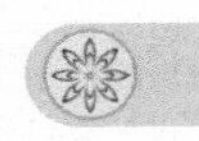

Grilled Steak with Creamed Spinach and Mushrooms

MAKES 4 SERVINGS

4 (3-ounce) boneless sirloin mini-steaks (or cut a 12-ounce steak into 4 pieces)

Salt and black pepper

2 tablespoons olive oil

2 cups chopped portobello or button mushrooms

4 cups baby spinach

$^{1}/_{2}$ cup heavy cream

Pinch of ground nutmeg

1. Preheat a grill pan over medium-high heat. Season the steaks with salt and pepper, then place in the grill pan and cook for 2 to 4 minutes on each side for medium-rare. Transfer the steaks to a platter and cover to keep warm.
2. Add the olive oil to a medium skillet over medium-high heat. When the oil is shimmering, add the mushrooms, stirring, for 3 to 4 minutes, or until lightly browned. Transfer to the platter with the steaks and spread on top. Cover again to keep warm.
3. Lower the heat for the skillet to medium and add the spinach and cream. Cook, stirring all the while, until the spinach has wilted and the cream has thickened a bit. Season to taste with some salt and the nutmeg.
4. Uncover the platter with the steak and mushrooms, and serve with the creamed spinach on the side.

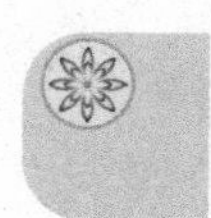

Slow Cooker Mushroom Stroganoff with Creamy Garlic Cauliflower Rice

MAKES 4 SERVINGS

FOR THE STROGANOFF

5 cups halved or quartered button mushrooms
6 garlic cloves, minced
1 medium yellow onion, thinly sliced
2 cups vegetable broth
4 teaspoons smoked paprika
2 tablespoons plain full-fat Greek yogurt
Salt and black pepper
1/4 cup chopped fresh parsley

FOR THE CAULIFLOWER RICE

1 medium cauliflower, trimmed and cut into florets
3 tablespoons olive oil
2 garlic cloves, minced
1 1/2 teaspoons salt
1 teaspoon black pepper
1/2 cup vegetable broth
4 tablespoons ghee (clarified butter) or unsalted butter
1/4 cup heavy cream

1. Make the stroganoff: Place the mushrooms, garlic, onion, broth, and paprika in a slow cooker and set to cook on high for 4 hours.
2. Open the cooker and stir in the yogurt. Season to taste with the salt and pepper. Cover the cooker and keep the stroganoff warm.
3. Make the cauliflower rice: Place the cauliflower florets in a food processor and process until they resemble grains of rice.
4. Heat a large saucepan over medium heat. Add the olive oil, then add the cauliflower rice, the garlic, salt, and pepper. Bring to a boil and cook for 3 minutes, stirring gently using a wooden spoon. Pour in the broth, cover the pot, then reduce the temperature to medium-low and simmer for 12 minutes, stirring gently and occasionally.
5. Stir in the ghee and cream, and simmer another 5 minutes, until creamy.
6. Serve the stroganoff with the creamy cauliflower rice.

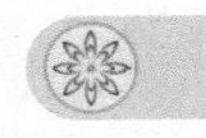

Blackened Tofu with Sesame Broccoli Slaw

MAKES 4 SERVINGS

1 (12-ounce) block extra-firm tofu, cubed

Herbs and seasonings of choice

4 tablespoons coconut oil

4 cups broccoli slaw

4 tablespoons sesame seeds

1. Place the tofu cubes in a medium bowl. Add the herbs and seasoning and rub to coat the cubes.
2. Place 2 tablespoons of the coconut oil in a large skillet over high heat. When melted, add the tofu and sauté for 3 to 4 minutes on each side, until blackened. Transfer to a bowl, cover, and keep warm.
3. Wipe out the skillet and then add the remaining 2 tablespoons coconut oil and place over medium-high heat. When the oil has melted, add the broccoli slaw and stir-fry until desired tenderness, about 2 minutes.
4. Spread the sautéed slaw on individual plates, then top with the blackened tofu. Sprinkle on the sesame seeds and serve.

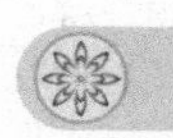

BBQ Tempeh, Greens, and Cauliflower Rice

MAKES 4 SERVINGS

$^1/_2$ cup Primal Kitchen BBQ sauce
$^1/_2$ cup fresh orange juice
2 $^1/_2$ tablespoons tamari
2 tablespoons apple cider vinegar
2 (8-ounce) packages tempeh
1 small head cauliflower (about 1 pound)
2 tablespoons ghee (clarified butter) or unsalted butter
$^1/_2$ medium yellow onion, finely diced
1 to 2 teaspoons garlic powder
$^1/_4$ teaspoon freshly grated nutmeg
Salt and black pepper
2 tablespoons olive oil
3 garlic cloves, minced
6 cups chopped fresh kale
1 tablespoon fresh lemon juice
2 tablespoons coconut oil
$^1/_2$ cup chopped fresh flat-leaf parsley
$^1/_2$ cup (2 ounces) grated Parmesan cheese
Roasted salted peanuts, coarsely chopped (optional)

1. In a small bowl, combine the barbecue sauce, orange juice, tamari, and vinegar. Pour the mixture into a shallow pan (an 8-inch square works great). Slice the tempeh in half horizontally, and then into triangles, for 16 triangles, each $^1/_4$ inch thick. Lay the tempeh in the marinade, spooning some sauce over the top. Let sit for at least 1 hour, and preferably overnight, flipping occasionally.
2. Cut the cauliflower into florets. In a food processor, pulse the florets just a few times to get the texture of rice.
3. Heat the ghee over medium heat in a large skillet, then add the onion and cook until translucent, about 4 minutes. Add the cauliflower, garlic powder, and nutmeg, then season to taste with salt. Sauté for 5 to 7 minutes to warm everything through, then cover and keep warm.
4. Place the olive oil in a large skillet over medium heat. When shimmering, add the garlic and sauté until fragrant, about 1 minute. Add the kale and sauté for 2 to 3 minutes, until wilted. Stir in the lemon juice and a pinch of salt and pepper.
5. Preheat an outdoor grill or heat a grill pan or cast-iron skillet on the stove to medium-high heat. Brush the grates or pan with the coconut oil. Drain the tempeh, reserving the marinade for cooking and serving. Grill or sauté the tempeh for 5 minutes on each side, brushing with the marinade occasionally.

6. Stir the parsley and Parmesan into the cauliflower rice and season with salt and pepper.
7. In large serving bowls, spoon a mound of the cauliflower rice, then add some of the tempeh and brush with the remaining marinade. Sprinkle on the peanuts and serve with the kale on the side.

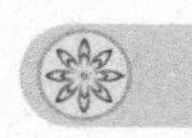

Veggie Cheese Enchiladas with Grain-Free Tortillas

MAKES 4 SERVINGS

FOR THE TORTILLAS

1 cup almond flour
1/4 cup coconut flour
2 teaspoons xanthan gum
1 teaspoon baking powder
1/2 teaspoon kosher salt
2 teaspoons fresh lime juice
1 large egg, lightly beaten
1 tablespoon water

FOR THE ENCHILADA SAUCE

1 1/2 cups no-added-sugar tomato sauce
1 cup vegetable broth
1 teaspoon apple cider vinegar
1 1/2 teaspoons chili powder
1 1/2 teaspoons smoked paprika
1 1/2 teaspoons ground cumin
1/2 teaspoon onion powder
1/2 teaspoon garlic powder
1 teaspoon salt

FOR THE FILLING

2 tablespoons avocado oil
1/3 small onion, diced
1 small bell pepper, cored and diced
1/2 small zucchini, diced
3 large eggs, lightly beaten
2 cups fresh spinach
1 tablespoon chili powder
1 1/2 teaspoons garlic salt
1 teaspoon onion powder
1/2 teaspoon ground cumin
1 1/2 cups (6 ounces) shredded cheddar cheese

1. Make the tortilla dough: Combine the almond flour, coconut flour, xanthan gum, baking powder, and salt in a food processor. Pulse for 5 seconds, until well blended.
2. With the food processor running, slowly pour in the lime juice, then add the egg, and finally the water. When the dough comes together and forms a ball, empty it onto a piece of plastic wrap. Knead the dough for a minute or two in your hands, then wrap in the plastic and place in the refrigerator to rest for 10 minutes.
3. Make the sauce: Place the tomato sauce, broth, vinegar, chili powder, paprika, cumin, onion powder, and garlic powder into a medium saucepan and stir to combine. Place over medium heat and bring to a near boil, then turn the heat to low and simmer until reduced by half or as thick as you like it, from 15 to 30 minutes.

4. Shape the tortillas: Divide the tortilla dough into 8 small balls, about 1 1/2 inches in diameter. Place a ball between 2 pieces of parchment or wax paper and roll out until about 1/8 inch thick; the tortilla should be 5 to 6 inches in diameter.
5. Heat a large cast-iron skillet over medium-high heat. When hot, add a tortilla and cook until slightly charred, about 20 seconds per side. Continue to roll out and cook the tortillas; while one tortilla is cooking, roll out the next. As the tortillas are finished cooking, stack them on a plate with pieces of parchment or wax paper between them. You'll need 8 tortillas for this recipe; you can freeze any remaining ones for future use.
6. Make the filling: Heat the avocado oil in a medium saucepan over medium heat, then add the onion and bell pepper. Sauté until the onion and pepper are softened, about 3 minutes. Stir in the zucchini and then add the eggs. Blend in the spinach, stir to combine, then when the spinach has wilted, add the chili powder, garlic salt, onion powder, and cumin. Reduce the heat and simmer, stirring, until the filling is blended and heated through.
7. Assemble the enchiladas: On a work surface, place one tortilla and then spoon on about 1/2 cup of the filling. Sprinkle on 1 1/2 tablespoons of the cheese, then roll up the tortilla, keeping the filling in place. Put the enchilada in a 13 by 9-inch baking dish and then continue to fill and roll the remaining 7 enchiladas.
8. Preheat the oven to 350°F. Pour the sauce over the enchiladas in the baking dish and sprinkle any remaining cheese on top. Bake for approximately 30 minutes, or until heated through, the sauce is bubbly, and the cheese is starting to brown on top. Serve while still hot.

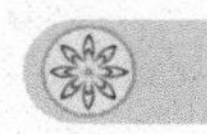

Spicy Edamame Bowl with Creamy Chili Sauce

MAKES 4 SERVINGS

FOR THE EDAMAME

2 ½ tablespoons toasted sesame oil
6 scallions, green and white parts divided and sliced
⅓ cup diced red onion
5 garlic cloves, minced
2 cups frozen edamame
1 teaspoon grated fresh ginger
1 tablespoon Sriracha or other hot sauce
1 (14-ounce) bag coleslaw mix
3 tablespoons tamari or soy sauce
1 tablespoon rice wine vinegar
⅛ to ¼ teaspoon ground white pepper
Salt
Black sesame seeds, for garnish

FOR THE CHILI SAUCE

¼ cup olive oil mayonnaise
1 tablespoon Sriracha or other hot sauce
Salt

1. Make the edamame: Heat the sesame oil in a large skillet over medium heat. When oil is hot, add the white parts of the scallions, the red onion, and garlic and sauté, stirring frequently, until the onion begins to soften, about 3 minutes.
2. Add the frozen edamame, ginger, and hot sauce and cook until edamame is heated through, about 3 minutes.
3. Add the coleslaw mix, tamari, vinegar, white pepper, and salt to taste, and stir until well combined. Cook, stirring regularly, until the cabbage is tender, about 5 minutes.
4. Meanwhile, make the chili sauce: In a small bowl, whisk together the mayonnaise and hot sauce. Season to taste with the salt.
5. Spoon the edamame mixture into serving bowls, then drizzle the chili sauce over. Garnish with the scallion greens and sprinkle with the black sesame seeds.

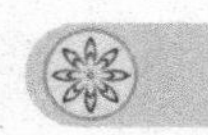

Celery Sticks with Almond Butter

MAKES 1 SERVING

- 2 tablespoons unsweetened almond butter
- 2 celery stalks, trimmed

Spread 1 tablespoon of the almond butter on each celery stalk.

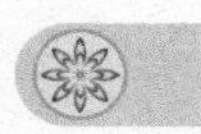

Carrots and Celery with Flaxseed and Almond Butter

MAKES 1 SERVING

- 2 tablespoons ground flaxseed
- 2 tablespoons unsweetened almond butter
- 10 baby carrots
- 2 celery stalks, cut in half crosswise

In a small bowl, mix the flaxseed with the almond butter until smooth. Use as a dip for the carrots and celery.

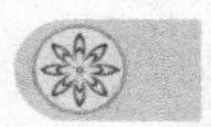

Caprese Bites

MAKES 24 SKEWERS

- 24 cherry tomatoes
- 24 fresh basil leaves
- 1 (8-ounce) package whole-milk fresh mozzarella balls
- 24 small skewers
- Olive oil

Thread a tomato, then a basil leaf folded in half, and then a mozzarella ball on each skewer. Place the skewers on a serving platter and drizzle with some olive oil. Figure 3 skewers per person.

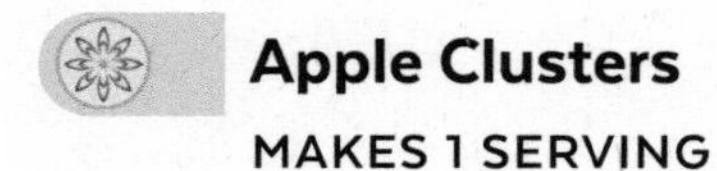

Apple Clusters

MAKES 1 SERVING

1 small apple, cored and sliced

2 tablespoons unsweetened almond butter

1 tablespoon chia seeds

1 tablespoon ground flaxseed

2 tablespoons unsweetened coconut flakes

1. Arrange the apple slices on a plate.
2. Combine the almond butter with the chia seeds and flaxseed in a microwave-safe small bowl and microwave on high for 15 to 30 seconds, until slightly melted.
3. Drizzle the almond butter mixture over the apple slices and top with the coconut flakes.

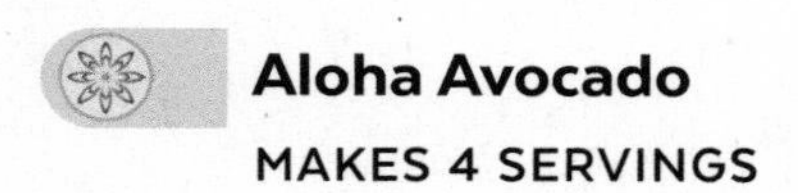

Aloha Avocado

MAKES 4 SERVINGS

2 ripe avocados

1 cup halved macadamia nuts

1/2 cup unsweetened coconut flakes

Halve the avocados and remove the pits. Cut the halves in half again, then fill the cavities with the nuts and coconut.

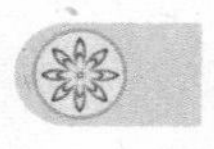

Pumpkin-Spiced Walnuts

MAKES 1 SERVING

1/4 cup whole walnuts

1 teaspoon avocado oil

1/2 teaspoon pumpkin pie spice

Place the walnuts in a small bowl. Drizzle with the avocado oil, then sprinkle with the pie spice. Mix well and then serve.

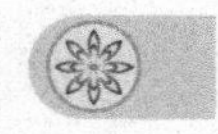

Avocado Crisps

MAKES 1 SERVING

1 avocado, halved, pitted, and chopped
1/4 cup grated Parmesan cheese
1 teaspoon fresh lemon juice
1/2 teaspoon garlic powder
1/2 teaspoon Italian seasoning

1. Preheat the oven to 325°F. Line a baking sheet with parchment paper.
2. In a medium bowl, mash the avocado until smooth. Add the cheese, lemon juice, garlic powder, and Italian seasoning. Mix well.
3. Spoon teaspoon-sized bits of the avocado mixture onto the baking sheet, spacing them evenly and spreading them thin. Bake for 15 to 18 minutes, or until the edges of the crisps have browned.

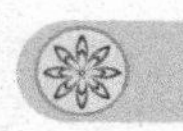

Cheese and Walnuts

MAKES 1 SERVING

1/4 cup walnut halves
1 cheese stick

Arrange the walnuts on a plate and add the cheese stick.

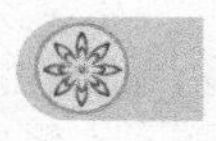

Cheesy Nuts

MAKES 1 SERVING

1 Babybel mini cheese round, wrapper removed
1/2 cup almonds

Arrange the cheese on a plate with the almonds.

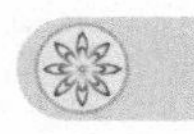

Everything-Bagel Cucumber Bites

MAKES 4 SERVINGS

1 medium cucumber

1 (4-ounce) package cream cheese

2 tablespoons salted butter

2 tablespoons plain full-fat Greek yogurt

4 teaspoons "everything bagel" seasoning

1. Cut the cucumber in half lengthwise.
2. In a small bowl, combine the cream cheese, butter, and yogurt, stirring until well blended.
3. Top the cucumber halves with the cream cheese mixture. Sprinkle the halves with the seasoning.
4. Cut the cucumber halves in half again to create 4 servings.

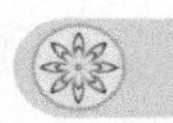

Crunchy Kale Chips with Pecans

MAKES 3 SERVINGS

Nonstick baking spray

1 large bunch fresh kale, stemmed and trimmed

2 tablespoons olive oil

1 tablespoon sea salt

3/4 cup chopped pecans

1. Preheat the oven to 350°F. Lightly grease a baking sheet with the baking spray or use a silicone mat.
2. Place the kale in a large zippered plastic bag. Add the olive oil, close the bag, and massage the leaves with the oil to coat well.
3. Spread out the kale on the baking sheet, flattening the leaves. Bake for 12 minutes, until leaves are crisp. Remove from the oven and sprinkle with the sea salt. Serve with the pecans.

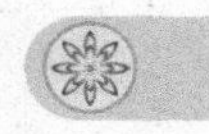

Creamy Avocado Dip

MAKES 1/2 CUP (1 SERVING)

1 avocado, halved and pitted, flesh scooped out

1 tablespoon avocado oil or olive oil mayonnaise

Juice of 1 lemon (3 tablespoons)

1 tablespoon chopped fresh cilantro

Combine the avocado, mayonnaise, lemon juice, and cilantro in a small bowl and mash with a fork until smooth. Serve the dip with your choice of veggie sticks or seeded crackers.

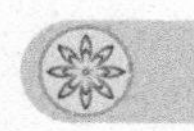

Easy Guacamole

MAKES ABOUT 2 CUPS (8 SERVINGS)

1/4 cup finely minced onion

3 ripe avocados

2 tablespoons fresh lime or lemon juice

1 large Roma (plum) tomato, seeded and diced

1/4 cup chopped fresh cilantro leaves and tender stems

1/2 teaspoon ground cumin

1/2 teaspoon salt

1. Place the onion in a small bowl, cover with warm water, and set aside to soften for 10 minutes.
2. Cut the avocados in half lengthwise and use a spoon to lift out the pit, then scoop out the flesh and place in a medium bowl.
3. Add the lime juice and mash the avocado with a fork until creamy but still chunky. Stir in the tomato, cilantro, and cumin. Drain the onion and add to the bowl along with salt to taste.
4. Taste the guacamole and adjust the seasonings. Serve with veggies of your choice, for dipping.

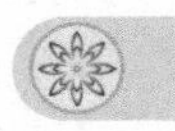

Herbed White Bean Dip

MAKES ABOUT $^{3}/_{4}$ CUP (2 SERVINGS)

$^{1}/_{2}$ cup cooked cannellini beans

$^{1}/_{2}$ lemon, juiced (about 1 $^{1}/_{2}$ tablespoons)

1 teaspoon grated lemon zest

2 tablespoons tahini or soy sauce

1 tablespoon olive oil

1 tablespoon chopped fresh dill

1 garlic clove

Place all of the ingredients in a food processor and process until smooth. Serve with veggies of your choice for dipping.

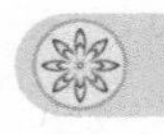

Herbed Cottage Cheese Dip with Cucumber

MAKES 2 SERVINGS

$^{1}/_{2}$ cup full-fat cottage cheese

1 tablespoon fresh lemon juice

$^{1}/_{2}$ teaspoon garlic powder

$^{1}/_{2}$ teaspoon onion powder

$^{1}/_{4}$ teaspoon black pepper

1 tablespoon chopped fresh dill

1 small cucumber, sliced

1. Place the cottage cheese, lemon juice, garlic powder, onion powder, pepper, and dill in a blender. Process until smooth.
2. Spoon the dip into a small bowl and dip the cucumber slices in it.

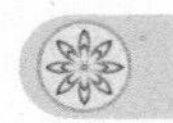

Veggie Slices with Italian Mayo Dip

MAKES 4 SERVINGS

1 cup olive oil mayonnaise

1 tablespoon Italian seasoning

2 large cucumbers, sliced

2 large carrots, sliced

8 asparagus, trimmed and cut into bite-sized pieces

8 radishes, trimmed and halved or quartered

1. In a small bowl, combine the mayonnaise and seasoning, stirring until well blended.
2. Arrange the cucumbers, carrots, asparagus, and radishes on platters and serve with the dip.

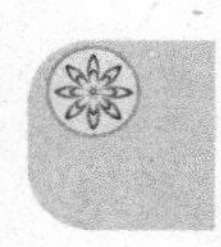

Marinated Olives, Chickpeas, and Vegetables with Thyme and Dill

MAKES 4 SERVINGS

2 large cucumbers, sliced

2 medium carrots, sliced

1 (15-ounce) can chickpeas, rinsed and drained

2 cups olives of choice

$^1/_2$ cup red wine vinegar

$^1/_4$ cup fresh thyme leaves

$^1/_4$ cup fresh dill

In a large bowl, combine the cucumbers, carrots, chickpeas, and olives. Pour in the vinegar and add the herbs. Stir well to combine the flavors, then cover and refrigerate for 15 minutes, until ready to serve.

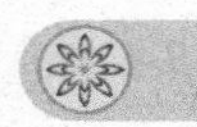

Cucumber, Tomato, and Feta Salad

MAKES 1 SERVING

1 medium cucumber, sliced

1 cup halved cherry tomatoes

$^1/_4$ small red onion, diced

1 garlic clove, minced

1 tablespoon olive oil

1 tablespoon red wine vinegar

2 tablespoons crumbled feta cheese

Place the cucumber, tomatoes, onion, and garlic in a small salad bowl. Drizzle on the olive oil and vinegar, and toss to dress the veggies. Scatter the feta on top.

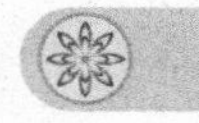

Turkey and Mayo Lettuce Wraps

MAKES 2 WRAPS (1 SERVING)

1 tablespoon olive oil mayonnaise

1 tablespoon red wine vinegar

1 tablespoon ground flaxseed

2 large lettuce leaves

2 ounces deli turkey slices

1 slice Swiss cheese

1. Combine the mayonnaise, vinegar, and flaxseed in a small bowl.
2. Lay the lettuce leaves on a flat surface and top each with some of the mayo, then layer on the turkey and cheese. Fold up and transfer to a serving plate.

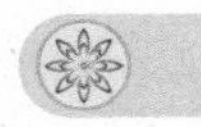

Hard-Boiled Egg with Avocado

MAKES 1 SERVING

1 hard-boiled large egg, shelled and split in half

$^1/_2$ avocado, peeled, pitted, and sliced

Place the egg halves on a serving plate and arrange the avocado slices alongside.

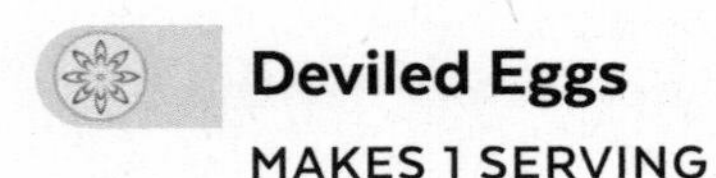

Deviled Eggs

MAKES 1 SERVING

2 hard-boiled large eggs

1 tablespoon avocado oil mayonnaise

1 tablespoon chia seeds

$^1/_4$ teaspoon ground turmeric

1 green bell pepper, cored and sliced

1. Peel the eggs, cut each in half, and gently remove the yolks.
2. Combine the yolks, mayonnaise, chia seeds, and turmeric in a small bowl. Spoon a little of the mayonnaise mixture into each egg white.
3. Place the stuffed eggs on a plate and accompany with the strips of green pepper.

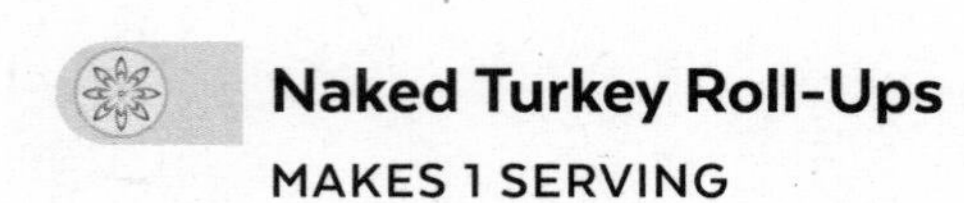

Naked Turkey Roll-Ups

MAKES 1 SERVING

2 ounces deli turkey slices

2 ounces Swiss cheese slices

1 tablespoon spicy brown mustard

Lay the turkey slices on a flat surface. Top with the cheese slices. Spread the mustard on top, then roll up.

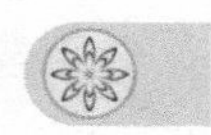

Edamame Mash Salad

MAKES 4 SERVINGS

1 $^1/_2$ cups frozen edamame
2 cups boiling water
2 garlic cloves
1 tablespoon lime juice
2 $^1/_2$ tablespoons avocado oil mayonnaise
2 tablespoons minced fresh cilantro
1 tablespoon minced fresh mint
1 tablespoon minced fresh dill
$^1/_4$ teaspoon stone-ground mustard
$^1/_4$ teaspoon salt
$^1/_4$ teaspoon ground black pepper
4 cups fresh spinach
1 cup shredded red cabbage

1. Put the edamame in a large bowl and pour the boiling water over it. Place a plate or lid on the bowl and let the edamame steam for 5 minutes. Drain the water and rinse the edamame until they are cool.
2. Place the edamame, garlic, lime juice, mayonnaise, herbs, mustard, salt, and pepper in a food processor and process just until the mash is blended but still has some texture. Transfer to a bowl and refrigerate until ready to assemble the salad.
3. Divide the spinach and cabbage evenly among 4 serving plates. Top with the edamame mash and serve.

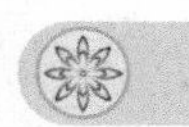

Pecans with Berries and Coconut

MAKES 1 SERVING

$^1/_4$ cup pecans
$^1/_4$ cup fresh blueberries
$^1/_4$ cup fresh strawberries
2 tablespoons unsweetened coconut flakes

Place the pecans, berries, and coconut in a small bowl and enjoy.

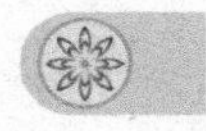

Pecans and Dark Chocolate

MAKES 1 SERVING

1 (1-ounce) piece of 70% or darker chocolate

1/4 cup pecans

Either melt the chocolate and dip the pecans in it or simply munch on the chocolate and pecans.

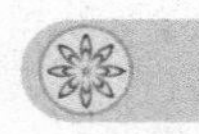

Raspberries with Pecans

MAKES 1 SERVING

1/2 cup fresh raspberries

1/4 cup pecans

Place the raspberries and pecans in a small bowl and enjoy.

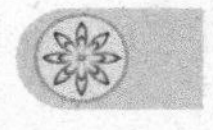

Nutty Berry Bowl

MAKES 1 SERVING

1/4 cup fresh strawberries, hulled and halved

1/4 cup fresh raspberries

1/4 cup fresh blackberries

1/4 cup fresh blueberries

2 tablespoons slivered almonds

Place the berries and nuts in a serving bowl and enjoy.

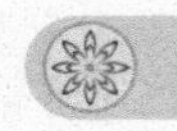

Tropical Berries

MAKES 1 SERVING

1/2 cup fresh blueberries

2 tablespoons unsweetened coconut flakes

Place the blueberries and coconut in a serving bowl and enjoy.

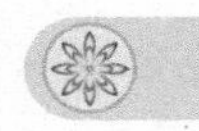

Strawberries with Chia Cream

MAKES 1 SERVING

- 1 cup halved fresh strawberries
- 2 tablespoons heavy cream
- 1 tablespoon chia seeds
- 1 tablespoon unsweetened coconut flakes

Place the strawberries in a small bowl. Drizzle on the cream, then sprinkle with the chia seeds and coconut flakes.

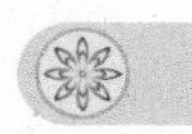

Pear Slices and Ricotta Cheese

MAKES 1 SERVING

- $^{1}/_{2}$ ripe medium pear, cored and sliced
- $^{3}/_{4}$ cup whole-milk ricotta (alternatively use dairy-free ricotta)
- Dash of ground cinnamon (optional)

Working quickly, so the pear doesn't oxidize, spread the slices on a plate. Spoon the ricotta alongside, then sprinkle the ricotta and pears with the cinnamon, if using.

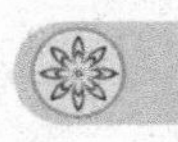

Chocolate Mocha Almonds with String Cheese

MAKES 6 SERVINGS

1 cup raw almonds (unsalted)
$^1/_2$ teaspoon olive oil
1 tablespoon unsweetened cocoa powder
1 teaspoon instant coffee granules
1 teaspoon Swerve powdered sugar
6 string cheese of choice

1. In a small nonstick skillet, toast almonds over low heat, stirring every couple of minutes, until they are fragrant, about 3 minutes. Add olive oil and stir to coat. Remove from heat.
2. Blend cocoa powder, coffee, and powdered sugar alternative in a high powered blender or food processor until the coffee granules are incorporated into a powder.
3. Pour almonds and cocoa mixture into a medium bowl and toss to coat evenly. Shake off excess. Spread over parchment or waxed paper to cool.
4. Store almonds in an airtight container at room temperature.

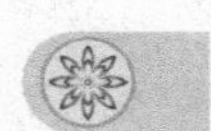

Blueberry Pie Smoothie

MAKES 1 SERVING

2 scoops collagen powder
1 scoop MCT powder or coconut oil
1 cup chopped fresh spinach
$^1/_2$ cup fresh blueberries
2 tablespoons chia seeds
2 tablespoons flax seeds
2 tablespoons unsweetened almond butter
$^1/_2$ teaspoon almond extract
Dash of grated nutmeg (optional)

Combine the powders, spinach, blueberries, seeds, and almond butter in a blender. Puree, then add the almond extract and nutmeg and pulse once more, until smooth.

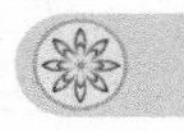

Mixed Berry Smoothie

MAKES 1 SERVING

$^1/_4$ cup halved fresh strawberries
$^1/_4$ cup fresh blackberries
$^1/_4$ cup fresh raspberries
$^1/_4$ cup plain full-fat Greek yogurt
1 cup baby spinach
1 tablespoon chia seeds
1 tablespoon ground flaxseed
Ice cubes

Place the berries, yogurt, spinach, chia seeds, and flaxseed in a blender and add a couple of ice cubes. Blend until smooth, adding a little water to thin to desired consistency, if needed.

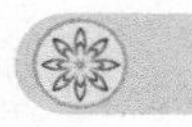

Raspberry Almond Smoothie

MAKES 1 SERVING

$^1/_2$ cup plain full-fat Greek yogurt
$^1/_2$ cup chopped fresh kale
$^1/_4$ cup fresh raspberries
1 tablespoon unsweetened almond butter
1 tablespoon chia seeds

Place all of the ingredients in a blender and process until smooth.

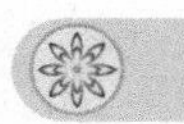

Peanut Butter Cup Smoothie

MAKES 1 SERVING

$^1/_4$ cup plain full-fat Greek yogurt
2 tablespoons unsweetened cocoa powder
2 tablespoons no-sugar-added peanut butter
1 tablespoon ground flaxseed
$^1/_2$ teaspoon vanilla extract
Ice cubes (optional)

Place the yogurt, cocoa, peanut butter, flaxseed, and vanilla in a blender. Add the ice cubes, if desired. Process until smooth.

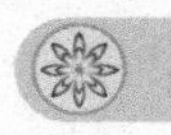

Peanut Butter–Mocha Smoothie

MAKES 1 SERVING

$^1/_2$ cup unsweetened almond milk
2 tablespoons chia seeds
2 tablespoons ground flaxseed
1 teaspoon unsweetened cocoa powder
2 tablespoons no-sugar-added peanut butter
$^1/_4$ teaspoon vanilla extract
$^1/_2$ peeled ripe banana, preferably frozen
1 shot (2 tablespoons) fresh espresso
$^1/_3$ cup crushed ice
Pinch of salt

Place the almond milk, chia seeds, flaxseed, cocoa, peanut butter, vanilla, banana, espresso, and ice in a high-powered blender. Process until smooth, then taste and season with salt.

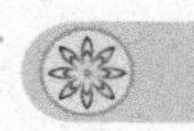

Green Almond Butter Smoothie

MAKES 1 SERVING

1 scoop vegan protein powder
1 cup almond milk
$^1/_2$ cup fresh blueberries
2 tablespoons almond butter
2 tablespoons ground flaxseed

Place all of the ingredients in a blender and process until smooth.

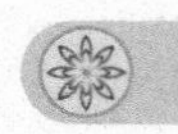

Vegan Cinnamon Roll Smoothie

MAKES 1 SERVING

2 scoops Carrington Farms Organic Coconut Protein Blend (other protein powders may alter the macro counts)
1 teaspoon cinnamon
$^1/_2$ teaspoon vanilla extract
2 tablespoons ground flax seeds
$^3/_4$ cup Kite Hill Unsweetened Almond Milk Yogurt (other dairy-free yogurt brands may impact macro counts)
1 cup unsweetened almond milk
1 cup ice cubes

Place all ingredients into a blender and pulse until smooth.

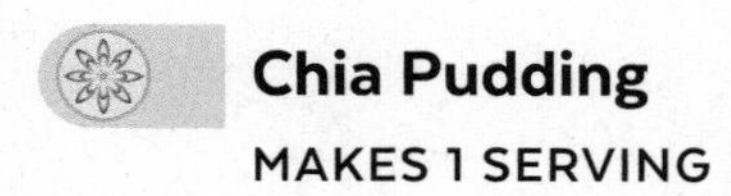

Chia Pudding

MAKES 1 SERVING

1 tablespoon flax seeds

2 tablespoons chopped pecans

Ground cinnamon

1/2 cup unsweetened coconut milk

1/4 cup chia seeds

In a small bowl, combine the flax seeds, pecans, and cinnamon to taste. Add the coconut milk slowly, stirring, until the ingredients are blended Sprinkle with the chia seeds and stir in gently. Cover and refrigerate 4 to 5 hours, or overnight, until the pudding has thickened.

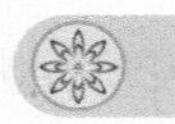

Coconut-Chia Pudding with Raspberries

MAKES 2 SERVINGS

1 (15-ounce) can unsweetened coconut milk

1/2 teaspoon vanilla extract

Pinch of stevia or monk fruit sweetener

1/4 teaspoon pumpkin pie spice

1/2 cup chia seeds

1/2 cup fresh raspberries

1. Place the coconut milk, vanilla, sweetener, and pumpkin pie spice into a medium bowl and stir well. Make sure all the coconut lumps get broken up and the liquid is smooth. Stir in the chia seeds and mix again.
2. Cover the bowl and refrigerate for 4 hours or more, or until thickened.
3. Spoon the pudding into individual bowls and top with the raspberries.

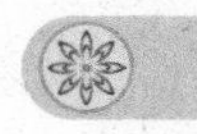

Coconut and Walnut Chia Pudding

MAKES 4 SERVINGS

4 cups unsweetened almond milk
4 tablespoons chia seeds
1/2 teaspoon stevia
1/2 teaspoon ground cinnamon
1/2 cup chopped walnuts
1/2 cup chopped pecans
1/4 cup sunflower seeds
1/4 cup unsweetened coconut flakes

In a medium bowl, combine the almond milk, chia seeds, stevia, and cinnamon in a bowl. Cover and refrigerate for 2 hours or overnight, until thickened. When ready to serve, spoon into individual bowls and top each with some of the nuts, sunflower seeds, and coconut flakes.

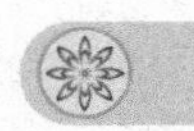

Peanut Butter and Chocolate Chia Pudding

MAKES 2 SERVINGS

FOR THE PUDDING

1/4 cup cacao powder or unsweetened cocoa powder
1 tablespoon Swerve sweetener
1/2 teaspoon ground cinnamon (optional)
Pinch of salt
1/2 teaspoon vanilla extract
1 1/2 cups unsweetened almond milk
1/2 cup chia seeds

FOR THE TOPPING

2 tablespoons no-sugar-added peanut butter
1/4 cup fresh raspberries

1. Make the pudding: Sift the cacao powder into a small bowl. Add the sweetener, cinnamon, salt, and vanilla, then whisk well. Add the almond milk gradually and whisk until a paste forms, then continue to whisk until smooth.
2. Stir in the chia seeds and whisk once more. Cover and refrigerate for 3 to 5 hours or overnight, until thickened. It may also be helpful to give the mixture an extra stir after it has been in the refrigerator for 30 to 45 minutes.
3. Make the topping: When ready to eat, melt the peanut butter in a small bowl in the microwave set on high for 20 to 30 seconds.
4. Spoon the pudding into serving bowls and top with a drizzle of the peanut butter and a sprinkling of the raspberries.

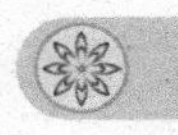

Chocolate Peanut Butter Yogurt

MAKES 1 SERVING

- $^1/_2$ cup plain full-fat Greek yogurt
- 1 tablespoon no-sugar-added peanut butter
- 1 tablespoon unsweetened cocoa powder
- 2 tablespoons chia seeds

Place the yogurt in a serving bowl and stir in the peanut butter, cocoa, and chia seeds.

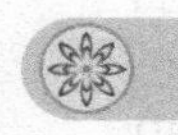

Vegan Yogurt Parfait

MAKES 1 SERVING

- $^1/_2$ cup plain unsweetened almond milk yogurt (such as Kite Hill)
- 1 scoop vanilla KOS Organic Plant Protein Powder (other brands may impact macro counts)
- 1 tablespoon ground flaxseed
- $^1/_3$ cup fresh blueberries
- $^1/_4$ cup pecans

Combine the yogurt, protein powder, and flaxseed in a small bowl. Top with the berries and pecans.

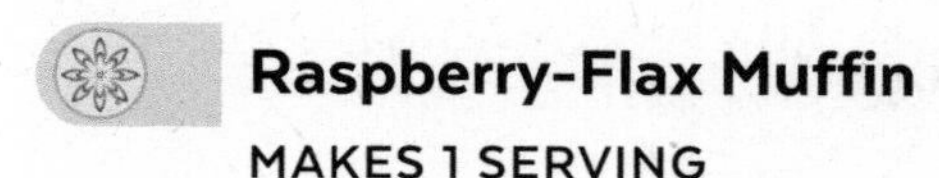

Raspberry-Flax Muffin

MAKES 1 SERVING

1 large egg
1 tablespoon coconut oil, melted
1 teaspoon vanilla extract
4 tablespoons ground flaxseed
1/2 teaspoon baking powder
1/4 teaspoon ground cinnamon
3 teaspoons monk fruit sweetener (with or without erythritol)
2 tablespoons fresh raspberries
1 tablespoon sugar-free dark chocolate chips
1 tablespoon whipped heavy cream

1. Place the egg, coconut oil, and vanilla in a small microwave-safe bowl. Stir well, then add the flaxseed, baking powder, cinnamon, and sweetener. Stir until well combined.
2. Add the raspberries and chocolate chips and mix again, then microwave on high for 90 seconds.
3. Let the "muffin" cool slightly, and then top with the whipped cream.

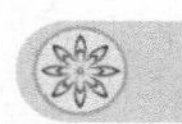

Chocolate-Cinnamon Apple Bites

MAKES ABOUT 6 MINI MUFFINS

Nonstick baking spray
1/2 cup unsweetened almond butter
1/4 cup unsweetened cocoa powder
1/4 cup coconut oil, melted
2 tablespoons unsweetened apple butter
Salt
1/2 teaspoon almond extract
Dash of ground cinnamon

1. Preheat the oven to 325°F. Grease a mini muffin pan with the baking spray.
2. Combine the almond butter, cocoa, coconut oil, and apple butter in a medium bowl. Add the almond extract and cinnamon, and stir to blend.
3. Spoon the batter into as many cups of the muffin tin as you have batter; fill the remaining cups with water. Bake for 10 minutes, or until a toothpick inserted in the center of a muffin comes out dry.
4. Pop the muffins out of the tin and serve 1 mini muffin per person.

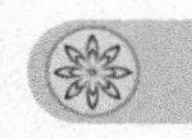

Chocolate Peanut Butter Mug Cake

MAKES 1 SERVING

- 1 tablespoon butter
- 1 large egg
- 1 tablespoon coconut flour
- 1 tablespoon stevia or monk fruit sweetener
- 1 tablespoon no-sugar-added peanut butter
- 1 tablespoon unsweetened cocoa powder
- $^1/_2$ teaspoon baking powder
- 2 tablespoons sugar-free dark chocolate chips

1. Place the butter in a microwave-safe large mug and microwave on high for 15 to 30 seconds, until melted.
2. Stir in the egg, coconut flour, stevia, peanut butter, cocoa, and baking powder and stir until well combined.
3. Add the chocolate chips and stir gently to distribute. Microwave on high for 60 seconds, then allow to cool slightly before serving.

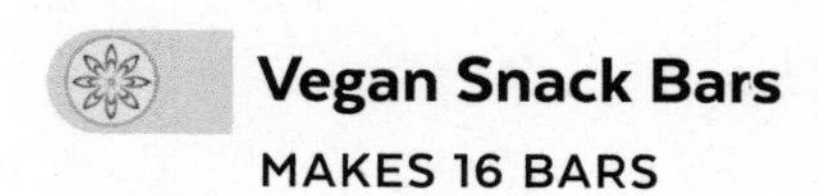

Vegan Snack Bars

MAKES 16 BARS

Nonstick cooking spray
½ cup almonds
½ cup walnut halves
½ cup macadamia nuts
½ cup pumpkin seeds
1 cup unsweetened shredded coconut
1 teaspoon ground cinnamon
½ cup no-sugar-added peanut butter
¼ cup coconut oil
2 teaspoons vanilla bean paste

1. Lightly grease a 6 by 10-inch baking pan with cooking spray and line with parchment paper.
2. Place the almonds, walnuts, macadamia nuts, and pumpkin seeds in a food processor and process until coarsely chopped. Transfer to a large bowl, then stir in the coconut and cinnamon.
3. Combine the peanut butter, coconut oil, and vanilla bean paste in a small saucepan and cook, stirring, over low heat for 3 to 5 minutes, or until melted and combined.
4. Pour the peanut mixture into the nuts mixture and stir until well combined. Press the mixture firmly into the prepared pan, smoothing the surface with the back of a spoon. Cover and refrigerate for 2 to 3 hours, or until firm. Cut into 16 bars, and figure 1 bar per serving.

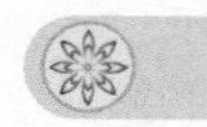

Chocolate Banana “Nice” Cream

MAKES 2 SERVINGS

2 ripe bananas, peeled
2 tablespoons unsweetened almond butter
¼ cup unsweetened almond milk
1 tablespoon unsweetened cocoa powder
3 tablespoons cacao nibs
1 tablespoon chia seeds
2 tablespoons ground flaxseed

Place all of the ingredients in a food processor and process until smooth. Pour into a freezer container and place in freezer to harden for several hours to overnight.

CHAPTER 10

The Galveston Diet for Life

Perhaps in the past you've been on a diet or nutritional plan, and you get to a point at which you want to just maintain your weight—or not gain back any you've lost. Not many plans offer a concrete way to do this, but the Galveston Diet does. The way it's done is to focus not only on just maintaining that weight loss but also on maintaining your new lifestyle. There's a difference. People who are the most successful at permanent weight loss are those who stick with the positive eating habits and lifestyle behaviors that have helped them reach their goals.

You've now lived the Galveston Diet for about a month. You've gotten the hang of the intermittent fasting and have incorporated into your shopping and cooking routines the idea of pairing anti-inflammatory nutrition with macronutrients in the right ratios, and of obtaining optimal micronutrients to avoid nutritional deficiencies. All three actions, especially when turned into positive habits, will help you stay successful from here on out.

Think of your new habits like paths through the woods. You form trails by walking them over and over, until there is a well-worn path.

Whenever you go for a walk in the woods, you'll then follow this easy, beautiful path instead of crashing your way through shrubs and brambles to get to your destination. The well-worn path feels good, too, and you'll want to walk it again and again. And so it is with your new, well-worn eating and lifestyle habits.

The Galveston Diet has been about restoring your health and wellness in an important phase of your life, one that will encompass 40 percent or more of that life! You've restored your body to a healthy weight and likely have healed a lot of health conditions. Naturally, you'll want to stay on that path!

So, the question is: How do you continue to live this lifestyle? The answer is to move into what I call "maintenance mode": you work these habits more and more firmly into your routine as you go along. You can, however, now make a few modifications to those routines—flexibility becomes the name of the game, once you have the core actions in place.

Continue Intermittent Fasting

By now, your body is used to intermittent fasting, so it should be an easy habit to maintain for a lifetime. I originally thought I'd do it only for a few months. But what started as an experiment actually turned into a way of life for me that's helped me take control of my weight, lower my inflammation, and feel amazing every day.

Although intermittent fasting is a modest way to shed pounds, its real power comes in keeping those pounds off. No more weight regain or yo-yo dieting. And I now make intermittent fasting part of my standard weight-loss maintenance advice to the women I counsel.

The bottom line is that for the first time we have a tool—a habit—that works for keeping weight off and inflammation levels low.

Science backs me up. In the past, when people lost weight they were generally advised to monitor and count calories so as to keep that weight off. But statistics tell us this method doesn't work: 95 percent of dieters regain their lost weight within a year, often with interest. And worse, 50 percent of the weight they lost was from fat and the other 50 percent was muscle mass.

In 2021, a group of researchers from the University of Kansas Medical Center conducted an interesting study involving intermittent fasting for weight-loss maintenance. They found that intermittent fasting was an effective alternative to counting calories as a way to prevent weight regain, and that it may just be a superior tool for helping people stay at a healthy weight.

Keep it up!

Eat Smarter and Live Better with Anti-Inflammatory Foods

By now, you realize that the food you eat plays a critical role in keeping inflammation at a low level, in improving your metabolism, in supporting weight loss, and in enhancing your health.

Because the Galveston Diet is really a pattern of eating versus a crash diet, it is among the most effective inflammation-fighting plans around. The key components from here on out are to eat a variety of foods (especially plants) that are high in antioxidants, phytochemicals, fiber, and healthy fats, as well as lean proteins and other nutrients. These foods and nutrients are the key proactive steps you can take to prevent disease, control your weight, and keep midlife symptoms from returning.

You now have even more flexibility in your food selections. On the maintenance program, you can expand your choices of anti-inflammatory foods. Now, for example, you can add more fruits, such as grapes, melons, papaya, pineapple, peaches, and virtually any other fresh fruit to your repertoire in increments of one or two servings a day.

You can also increase your intake of carbohydrates with an extra serving or two of starchy carbs such as sweet potatoes, winter squash, various root vegetables, and whole grains. All these foods have enormous anti-inflammatory power. Just be sure to track your carb macros to make sure they match your maintenance allowance (see page 229).

Remember, the Galveston Diet is a forever plan that's all about choice—your choice—to eat well and live well. And as I've pointed out, it has nothing to do with willpower and everything to do with learning about your body and reinforcing the behaviors for life that will create the healthiest version of you.

Anti-inflammatory foods are a huge part of all this. They cut your risk of long-term disease—so eat them every day! Inflammation, however, can come back quickly if you revert to the wrong foods. So, you've got to fight off inflammation for good with the right nutrition.

Change Up Your Fuel Ratios

As your waist-hip ratio, weight, and other markers of good health improve, you can begin to change your macro ratios over the course of a few weeks. What this means is that you can now eat more good carbs and less fat, while sticking to a moderate amount of protein.

This involves readjusting your macros—in other words, you'll make a shift in the percentages of carbohydrate and fat. Once you've reached a point at which you're healthier, feel great, and like your size, you no longer need to follow a macro formula that puts your body in a fat-burning mode. You can stabilize everything with a macro adjustment.

Why is this the case? Because now, everything should be rocking. Your hormones are better regulated, your metabolism is healthier, and you have more energy. Your body can now handle a different percentage of macros.

You'll still continue to choose anti-inflammatory foods that honor your body—and more of them. You'll still refocus your fuel but with different macros, and you'll do this gradually. "Gradual" is the name of the game here. It moves the needle slowly, and as a result, it makes changes far more likely to stick.

Here's how to do this:

- Start with one or more weeks at 60 percent fat, 20 percent protein, and 20 percent carbohydrates.
- Progress to additional weeks at 50 percent fat, 20 percent protein, and 30 percent carbohydrate.
- Stabilize over the long term at 40 percent fat, 20 percent protein, and 40 percent carbohydrates.

Of course, it's important to continue to track your macronutrients as you make these adjustments. Take your time and be sure to pay attention to how your body feels with these adjustments—and be patient. Each new adjustment may take a few weeks to become a habit.

Monitor your weight, too. On maintenance, go with weekly weigh-ins or weigh a few times each week. People who have successfully kept weight off and are a part of the National Weight Control Registry—the largest study of people who have been successful at long-term weight loss—maintain their weight by stepping on the scale about once a week.

Don't forget to monitor your non-scale changes as well. Keep track of your waist-to-hip ratio, as discussed earlier. As you continue adding more foods back into your diet, it's important to recognize if a reintroduced food is causing any inflammation or discomfort. If so, consider reducing the amount of that food or eliminating it from your diet.

Don't be alarmed over a 5-pound weight gain; that's usually normal. But if you find weight creeping back higher than that, or if your waist-to-hip ratio is not what it should be, an alarm bell should sound. That's a signal to rein yourself in by returning briefly to the 70 percent fat, 20 percent protein, and 10 percent carbohydrate ratios.

As you adjust your ratios on maintenance, consider these tips:

- All the recipes in this book can be modified in some way to better suit the maintenance macros.

- Replace lower-carb vegetables with whole grains, legumes, and starchier squashes and fruits.
- Reduce the amount of healthy fats enjoyed at each meal and snack time. An example would be eating 1/2 avocado versus a whole or using 1 tablespoon olive oil versus 2 tablespoons.
- Continue to select anti-inflammatory foods. Maintenance does not mean returning to tons of processed/refined carbs! My personal rule of thumb is that if a food is made in nature and doesn't require a label, it's a thumbs-up! But if a food is made in a factory, does not look like a naturally occurring food (grains don't grow in the shape of a Cheerio, for instance), or is a "food-like substance" with flavors created by a scientist (like some chips), that's a big thumbs-down.

When purchasing condiments, it's essential to review the ingredients and avoid added sugars and inflammatory ingredients whenever possible.

The Joy of Change

Amazing things happen when you do the Galveston Diet for life!

At age 43, Valerie had a complete hysterectomy. Although she had never had a weight problem, she noticed her weight creeping up over the years. By age 50, she had gained noticeable menopausal weight, reaching 134 pounds on her very small frame, especially around her middle.

"I had a belly pooch that I've never had in my life. I am curvy and love that, but not "poochy." Anyway, I lost 6 pounds in two weeks! As of right now, I'm down to my goal weight of 120 pounds.

"Most of all, I no longer experience bloating, constipation and have eliminated added sugar from my diet. Also, my pooch is gone. I feel wonderful! All this [was] done with no pills, gimmicks, or unrealistic eating that no person can maintain."

Then there is Laurie, who was going through menopause. After six weeks on the program, she lost 12 pounds, along with seeing several other positive changes. "I've also noticed that my hips no longer ache after driving or sitting for an extended period," she said. "This relief is amazing for me since this pain had become increasingly worse and made me wonder if I might need a hip replacement. I'm a very busy midwife in Michigan, and I plan to work for quite a few more years, as long as I feel healthy. And I feel so healthy after eating the way the program has taught me."

After Mayra got her blood work back recently, she was elated. "I'm no longer prediabetic or have borderline high cholesterol. As I continue to do the program and exercise, I'll drop the remaining weight, but the best part is that I have no menopause symptoms at all. They were mild before, but nothing now."

And Debbie is an intermittent fasting "lifer." "I followed the eating plan and practiced the 16:8 intermittent fasting schedule. I lost 77 pounds and have never felt better. I wish I had known about intermittent fasting earlier in my life because it has helped me keep my weight off. In the past, I always yo-yoed in weight, but not anymore."

Maintenance Meal Plans

Here are some examples of what would constitute a meal plan when you're on maintenance. I've provided sample two-day menus for conventional and vegetarian meals. Mostly, these sample menus reference the maintenance-adjusted recipes that follow, but also include a few earlier recipes in this book.

Conventional Menu

DAY 1

MEAL 1: MARY CLAIRE'S PARFAIT (PAGE 173)

Snack 1: Nutty Banana Toast (page 244)

MEAL 2: MEATLOAF WITH MASHED CAULIFLOWER AND BAKED SWEET POTATO (PAGE 236)

Snack 2: Date Night (page 244)

Macros: Fat: 43%, Protein: 21%, Net Carbs: 36%, Fiber: 29g

DAY 2

MEAL 1: MINI-AVOCADO "FOR LIFE" TOAST (PAGE 237)

Snack 1: Chickpea and Tomato Salad (page 245)

MEAL 2: LEMON-CAPER CHICKEN WITH FARRO (PAGE 238)

Snack 2: Summer Fruit Salad (page 245)

Macros: Fat: 40%, Protein: 24%, Net Carbs: 36%, Fiber: 34g

Vegetarian Menu

DAY 1

MEAL 1: TOFU IN PEANUT SAUCE WITH BROWN RICE (PAGE 239)

Snack 1: 2 hard-boiled eggs

MEAL 2: VEGAN PROTEIN LOWER-FAT SALAD (PAGE 240)

Snack 2: Cinnamon Baked Apple with Raisins (page 246)

Macros: Fat: 47%, Protein: 16%, Net Carbs: 37%, Fiber: 27g

DAY 2

MEAL 1: OAT CAKES WITH ALMOND BUTTER AND BLUEBERRIES (PAGE 242)

Snack 1: Green Almond Butter Smoothie (page 220)

MEAL 2: SLOW COOKER MUSHROOM STROGANOFF WITH CREAMY BROWN RICE (PAGE 243)

Snack 2: Lemon-Ricotta Dip with Pear Slices (page 246)

Macros: Fat: 48%, Protein: 16%, Net Carbs: 36%, Fiber: 31g

Maintenance Versions of Galveston Diet Recipes

Meal 1 and Meal 2 Recipes

Following are seven maintenance versions of recipes included earlier in *The Galveston Diet*. All include small changes that reflect the shift in your ratios for maintenance eating.

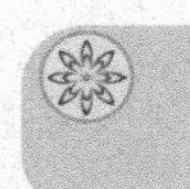

Meatloaf with Mashed Cauliflower and Baked Sweet Potato

In this maintenance version of the meatloaf recipe on page 198, I upped the carbs by swapping out almond flour for oat flour (which is higher in carbohydrates). Serve a slice of this meatloaf with a small baked sweet potato, and you've plated up a delicious meal of good carbs with lots of anti-inflammatory benefits.

MAKES 6 SERVINGS

- 2 tablespoons olive oil
- $^1/_4$ cup chopped onion
- 1 $^1/_2$ pounds lean, grass-fed ground beef
- 1 cup oat flour
- 2 large eggs
- $^1/_3$ cup no-sugar-added tomato sauce
- $^1/_2$ cup grated Parmesan cheese
- $^1/_2$ teaspoon salt
- $^1/_2$ teaspoon black pepper
- $^1/_2$ teaspoon garlic powder
- 6 small sweet potatoes
- 2 cups mashed cauliflower (from frozen or homemade)
- 6 tablespoons ($^3/_4$ stick) salted butter

1. Preheat the oven to 350°F.
2. Heat the olive oil in a small skillet, add the onion, and sauté until it turns translucent, about 3 minutes.
3. In a large bowl, combine the ground beef, sautéed onion, oat flour, eggs, tomato sauce, cheese, salt, pepper, and garlic powder. Shape the mixture into a firm oval loaf.
4. Place the loaf in a shallow baking pan or loaf pan, and bake for 1 hour. When the loaf has been baking for about 15 minutes, poke the sweet potatoes with a fork and place on the oven rack alongside the pan or on another rack of the oven.
5. Meanwhile, prepare the mashed cauliflower according to package instructions.
6. Carefully remove the loaf from the pan, discarding the surrounding fat, and transfer to a serving platter. Also, test the sweet potatoes and, if soft, remove from the oven.
7. Slice the loaf for serving, place the slices on plates, and accompany with portions of the mashed cauliflower and a sweet potato. If desired, top the servings of cauliflower with generous pats of butter.

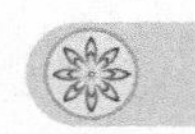

Mini-Avocado "For Life" Toast

Here's an example of how you can modify a simple recipe to supply a little less fat. To change the full recipe on page 175, I simply cut back the olive oil and used half an avocado instead of a whole one.

MAKES 1 SERVING

$^1/_2$ teaspoon olive oil
2 large eggs
2 slices sprouted-grain bread (such as Food For Life brand)
$^1/_2$ avocado, pit removed, sliced
Salt and black pepper
Red pepper flakes (optional)

1. Heat the olive oil over medium heat in a large skillet until shimmering. Add the eggs and cook to your preferred style, either fried or scrambled, about 3 minutes.
2. Meanwhile, toast the bread to desired doneness.
3. Place the toast on a serving plate. Add the avocado slices, then add the eggs and season to taste with salt and pepper. Sprinkle with the red pepper flakes, if using. Serve at once.

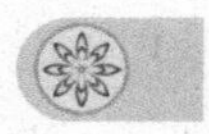

Lemon-Caper Chicken with Farro

On maintenance, you can begin to enjoy more grains so as to slightly increase your carbohydrates. This maintenance version of Lemon Chicken with Capers (page 195) includes farro, a high-fiber, high-protein whole-grain wheat that is yummy.

MAKES 4 SERVINGS

- 4 skinless, boneless chicken breast halves (about 1 pound)
- Salt and black pepper
- 4 tablespoons ghee (clarified butter) or olive oil
- 2 lemons, 1 juiced and 1 sliced
- 1 garlic clove, sliced
- 2 tablespoons drained capers
- 1 large onion, sliced
- 4 cups trimmed green beans
- 1/4 cup slivered almonds, toasted
- 4 cups cooked farro, warm
- 2 tablespoons salted butter

1. Pat the chicken pieces dry and season to taste with salt and pepper.
2. In a large skillet over medium-high heat, add 1 tablespoon of the ghee and, when shimmering, add the chicken pieces. Cook, flipping once, for 8 to 10 minutes, until cooked through. Transfer the chicken to a plate. Cover and keep warm.
3. To the skillet, add the lemon juice, 1 tablespoon of the ghee, the garlic, and capers and bring to a simmer over medium-high heat. Add the lemon slices, then return the chicken to the skillet and reduce the heat. Simmer the chicken for 5 minutes.
4. In another medium skillet over medium heat, warm the remaining 2 tablespoons ghee. When shimmering, add the onion and beans, and cook until the onion is translucent and the beans are fork-tender, about 5 minutes.
5. Toss the slivered almonds into the beans and stir to combine.
6. Arrange the chicken on a serving platter and accompany with the onion and beans. Spoon the farro alongside and top with pats of butter.

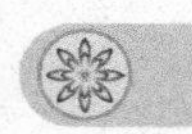

Tofu in Peanut Sauce with Brown Rice

Here's an Asian-inspired vegetarian dish but without all the sugary sauce. This maintenance version of Tofu in Peanut Sauce (page 187) supplies extra carbs with the addition of brown rice, which is rich in fiber and full of magnesium.

MAKES 4 SERVINGS

- 1 (14-ounce) square firm tofu
- 1/4 cup no-added-sugar peanut butter
- 2 tablespoons tamari
- 2 tablespoons water
- 3 tablespoons Swerve sweetener
- 1 teaspoon toasted sesame oil
- 1/2 teaspoon red pepper flakes
- 1 tablespoon grated fresh ginger
- 2 1/4 cups chopped fresh broccolini
- 1 tablespoon coconut oil
- 4 cups steamed brown rice, warm

1. Sandwich the tofu between 2 paper towels and 2 plates. Place a heavy item like a can on the top plate, and press the tofu for at least 30 minutes. The cut the tofu into 1/2-inch cubes; you should have about 1 1/2 cups.
2. In a small bowl, combine the peanut butter, tamari, water, and sweetener. Add the sesame oil, red pepper flakes, and ginger.
3. Steam or boil the broccolini until tender, about 5 minutes. Keep warm.
4. Heat the coconut oil in a large skillet over medium heat and when melted, add the tofu and cook for 10 to 15 minutes, occasionally turning, until lightly browned.
5. Stir in the sauce and blend well. Place the brown rice in serving bowls and spoon the tofu mixture over. Serve with the broccolini on the side.

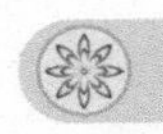

Vegan Protein Lower-Fat Salad

Here's another example of how you can slightly reduce the fat in a recipe—by cutting back on olive oil and tahini, and using half an avocado rather than a whole. This is the maintenance version of Vegan Protein Salad (page 181).

MAKES 2 SERVINGS

FOR THE TEMPEH

2 tablespoons balsamic vinegar
1 tablespoon tamari or soy sauce
1 tablespoon pure maple syrup
½ teaspoon garlic powder
Pinch of salt and black pepper
½ block tempeh (about 4 ounces), cut into cubes

FOR THE TOFU

½ block medium or firm tofu (about 5 ounces), cut into cubes
½ teaspoon garlic powder
1 tablespoon tamari or soy sauce
Pinch of salt and black pepper

FOR THE SALAD

1 cup chopped and steamed broccoli
2 cups lightly chopped fresh arugula
1 cup diced cucumber
1 avocado, pitted and chopped
4 tablespoons hemp seeds
2 teaspoons tahini
1 teaspoon olive oil
Fresh lemon juice

1. Make the tempeh: Mix the balsamic vinegar, tamari, maple syrup, garlic powder, and salt and pepper in a shallow dish. Add the tempeh and let soak for at least 2 hours and up to overnight.
2. When ready, preheat the oven to 400°F. Either spray a small baking dish with nonstick cooking spray or line it with a silicone baking mat.
3. Transfer the tempeh cubes to the baking dish and bake the tempeh for 20 minutes. Toss the tempeh cubes with a with a bit of the leftover marinade, if desired. Keep the oven turned on.
4. Make the tofu: Toss the tofu cubes with the garlic powder, tamari, and salt and pepper and bake at 400°F for 30 minutes, until lightly browned. (If desired, bake it at the same time as you bake the tempeh.)

5. Assemble the salad: Place the broccoli, arugula, cucumber, and avocado in a large salad bowl. Add the tempeh and tofu cubes, and mix well. Sprinkle on the hemp seeds. Drizzle on the tahini and olive oil, then toss to coat everything well with the dressing. Finish the salad with a spritz of fresh lemon juice and serve.

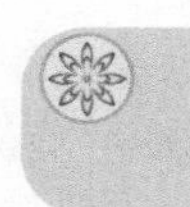

Vegetarian Oat Cakes with Almond Butter and Blueberries

This delicious breakfast or brunch dish substitutes oat flour for the ground flaxseed in the Flaxseed Pancakes (page 176). Oat flour is slightly higher in carbs and is a great source of fiber, vitamins, and minerals. In fact, try using oat flour rather than white flour to bump up the good carbs in any of your recipes.

MAKES 4 SERVINGS

1 cup oat flour
4 large eggs, lightly beaten
$^1/_3$ cup unsweetened almond milk (or other milk), or more as needed
2 teaspoons fresh lemon juice
1 teaspoon baking soda
1 teaspoon vanilla extract
1 teaspoon ground cinnamon
$^1/_8$ teaspoon salt
$^1/_2$ tablespoon coconut oil
4 tablespoons unsweetened almond butter
2 cups frozen blueberries

1. In a large bowl, combine the oat flour, eggs, almond milk, lemon juice, baking soda, vanilla, cinnamon, and salt. If the mixture is too thick, add more almond milk or water to achieve a batter consistency.
2. Heat a large skillet over medium heat and add the coconut oil. When melted and hot, pour about $^1/_4$ cup of the batter for each oat cake and gently spread it with a spoon. Let cook on one side for 2 to 3 minutes or until the edges begin to firm and bubbles appear, then flip and cook on the opposite side for another 2 to 3 minutes. Keep the cooked oat cakes warm on a covered plate while you make any remaining cakes with the remaining batter.
3. Meanwhile, melt the almond butter in a small bowl in the microwave. Place the frozen blueberries in a medium bowl and microwave until they are no longer frozen, have warmed slightly, and become juicy.
4. Place the oat cakes on serving plates, drizzle with the melted almond butter, and sprinkle with the blueberries.

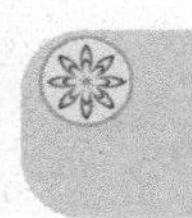

Slow Cooker Mushroom Stroganoff with Creamy Brown Rice

In the recipe on page 200, the stroganoff is served with cauliflower rice. Here, the stroganoff is accompanied with brown rice, a terrific source of quality carbs and fiber. I've also increased the yogurt and parsley and decreased the amount of fat.

MAKES 4 SERVINGS

FOR THE STROGANOFF

5 cups halved or quartered button mushrooms

6 garlic cloves, minced

1 medium yellow onion, thinly sliced

2 cups vegetable broth

4 teaspoons smoked paprika

2 tablespoons plain full-fat Greek yogurt

Salt and black pepper

1/2 cup chopped fresh parsley

FOR THE CREAMY RICE

3 tablespoons olive oil

4 cups cooked brown rice

2 garlic cloves, minced

1 1/2 teaspoons salt

1 teaspoon black pepper

1/2 cup vegetable broth

2 tablespoons ghee (clarified butter) or unsalted butter

2 tablespoons heavy cream

1. Make the stroganoff: Place the mushrooms, garlic, onion, broth, and paprika in a slow cooker and set to cook on high for 4 hours.
2. Open the cooker and stir in the yogurt. Season to taste with the salt and pepper. Cover the cooker and keep the stroganoff warm.
3. Make the creamy rice: Heat a large saucepan over medium heat and add the olive oil. When hot, add the brown rice, garlic, salt, and pepper and cook for 3 minutes, stirring gently with a wooden spoon. Pour in the vegetable broth, cover, and reduce the heat to medium-low. Simmer for 12 minutes, stirring gently and occasionally.
4. Stir in the ghee and cream, and stir while simmering for another 5 minutes.
5. Serve the stroganoff with the creamy garlic brown rice.

SNACK RECIPES

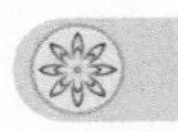

Nutty Banana Toast

Bananas are one of the fruits you can enjoy on the Galveston Diet. They are a great source of potassium and electrolytes, and are a good way to increase your carbohydrate macro.

MAKES 1 SERVING

2 slices sprouted-grain bread (such as Food For Life)

1 tablespoon unsweetened almond butter

1 medium banana, sliced

Ground cinnamon (optional)

Toast the bread to desired doneness. Spread the toast with the almond butter, then lay on the banana slices. If desired, sprinkle with the cinnamon, then serve.

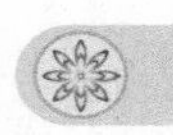

Date Night

Dates are a delicious source of natural sweetness. Plus, they are a good source of potassium, magnesium, and iron. Dates also rate high on indices that measure antioxidant activity. So, coupled with some dark chocolate, the dates here will give you a big punch of antioxidants and have welcome anti-inflammatory benefits.

MAKES 1 SERVING

1 (1-ounce) square 70% or darker chocolate

2 medjool dates, pitted

Place the chocolate in a small bowl and microwave on low until melted, 2 to 3 minutes. Dip or roll the dates in the melted chocolate.

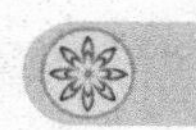

Chickpea and Tomato Salad

When you prepare recipes with legumes like chickpeas, you're getting a lot of good carbs, protein, and fiber all in one dish. This snack is easy to fix and packed with benefits.

MAKES 1 SERVING

1 cup canned chickpeas, drained and rinsed

1 cup halved or quartered grape tomatoes

2 extra-large pitted black olives, sliced

1 tablespoon minced onion

1 tablespoon balsamic vinegar

In a medium bowl, combine the chickpeas, grape tomatoes, olives, and onion. Drizzle on the vinegar and allow the mixture to sit for 10 to 15 minutes before eating.

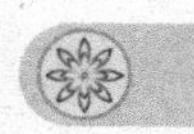

Summer Fruit Salad

On maintenance, you get to eat more fresh fruit. One way to make that happen is to prepare a fruit salad like this one, in which you get a variety of colorful fruits, all rich in antioxidants.

MAKES 1 SERVING

1 medium banana, sliced

$^1/_2$ cup sliced fresh strawberries

$^1/_2$ cup cubed fresh watermelon

Combine the banana, strawberries, and watermelon in a medium bowl and enjoy.

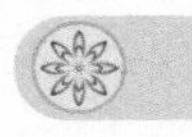

Cinnamon Baked Apple with Raisins

One easy way to up your carb intake is to combine fruits in a recipe like this one. Here, an apple is paired with raisins, both high in good carbs, plus with lots of fiber.

MAKES 1 SERVING

1 teaspoon salted butter

¼ cup raisins of choice

1 medium apple, cored

¼ teaspoon ground cinnamon

Place the butter and raisins in the cavity of the apple, then sprinkle with the cinnamon. Place in a small bowl and microwave the apple on medium for 1 to 2 minutes, or until softened slightly.

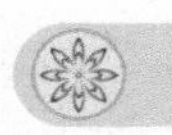

Lemon-Ricotta Dip with Pear Slices

Pears are among the highest fiber fruits you can eat. Enjoy them with this delicious dip.

MAKES 4 SERVINGS

1 cup whole-milk ricotta

1 lemon, juiced

2 tablespoons olive oil

2 tablespoons chopped fresh basil

4 pears, any variety, split, cored, and sliced

Place the ricotta, lemon juice, olive oil, and basil in a small bow. Mix well, then serve with the pear slices.

Eating Out

The Galveston Diet is so versatile, with so many different foods, that you're not doomed to cook all your meals at home; it just means you'll want to make the right selections when you do dine out.

Increasingly, restaurants are serving foods that are healthy and fresh. Many menus include lots of grilled meats and fish, fresh vegetables of all types, and many other healthy ingredients. As a result, it's not difficult to eat out while you're living the Galveston Diet lifestyle.

As a rule of thumb, just remember to select menu items based on the general eating pattern of lean protein, vegetables (like a side salad and/or low-carb veggies), and a healthy starch, such as a small sweet potato or a small portion of brown rice.

For example, select your entree from lean meat (such as a small sirloin or filet mignon), broiled or roasted chicken or turkey, or baked, grilled, or poached fish. Then choose from the vegetable sides or salads with vinaigrette dressing, and you're all set.

Don't be afraid to ask for substitutions or additions. Now, more than ever, restaurants are happy to accommodate special requests, such as holding the fries and doubling the vegetables. The foods that don't align with your goals will not go to waste, and they won't be staring up at you, tempting you!

As healthy as the dining options are becoming, the portions at most restaurants are far larger than we'd dish up for ourselves at home. So, remember, when you feel full, you don't have to finish it all. Take the rest home in a doggie bag for another meal.

Here are some specific tips for dining out that should be helpful when living the Galveston Diet lifestyle.

Sandwich shops and burger restaurants. A lot of these establishments will prepare burgers and other protein-filled sandwiches on giant lettuce leaves rather than on buns—if you ask. This choice is a great way to shave processed carbohydrates off your meal.

Bowls and salad entrees. I love to see these on the menu, especially bowls that often replace burritos or tacos on Southwestern or Mexican menus. You can ask for a bowl (or salad) made of protein, lettuce, legumes, a little cheese, salsa, and guacamole, for example. Any salad can be a great entree when piled with grilled chicken or shrimp, legumes, and sliced avocado. Getting nuts into the mix can be challenging, but many restaurants offer grilled meat or chicken that can be served with a side salad, rice, or a small cup of black beans or charro beans. Some Mexican restaurants even offer high-fiber tortillas that can be filled with meat or beans.

Asian restaurants. These offer a variety of meats, seafood, and veggies for a stir-fry. The key here is to ask for the dish with a light sauce and with a little bit of brown rice on the side. Black bean sauce might be a healthy bet, for example. Other good menu choices include steamed or lightly stir-fried vegetables; be sure to ask for extra veggies with any dish.

Also, moo shu vegetable or chicken or moo goo gai pan is usually loaded with vegetables like cabbage, mushrooms, carrots, water chestnuts, bamboo shoots, and sometimes cashews, and flavored with ginger and garlic. Try having a broth-based Asian soup for starters. It will really fill you up.

Steakhouses. Traditional options like steak, grilled chicken or fish, side salads, and fresh veggies are easy to order here. Just make sure that no sugary glazes or sauces come with your dish. Or, see if your protein can be topped with sautéed mushrooms. Many of these places also offer entree salads that can be made Galveston Diet friendly.

Greek and Mediterranean restaurants. Opt for the delicious and healthy items sure to be on these menus, like grilled meats and Greek salads. For a vegetarian dish, order hummus with sliced cucumbers for dipping (always a better choice than pita bread).

Italian. Italian food isn't all about the pasta! Indeed, in Italy itself, many regions don't eat much of it at all. When you're eating out at an Italian restaurant, look at the *secondi* part of the menu—that's where the non-pasta entrees are usually hiding. Structure your meal around a lean protein like steak, chicken, or fish. Avoid the bread and enjoy plenty of fresh vegetables dressed with olive oil.

Indian. Tandoori chicken is always a sure bet here. Have some veggies on the side or a small serving of curried chickpeas. This cuisine is typically prepared with lots of anti-inflammatory spices, too.

Pizza. I've noticed lately that many pizza restaurants are catering to the low-carb crowd by offering pizza made with cauliflower crusts. If you find a place that offers a crust like this, pile it high with veggies like peppers, onions, and mushrooms. Don't forget some olives for a little extra fat.

Breakfast. If you're eating breakfast out (on a break during your morning fast), stick to eggs, a little side of fruit, and maybe some turkey bacon. Veggie omelets are a great choice, too.

Other Lifestyle Guidelines

As the three actions described in *The Galveston Diet* become everyday habits, you'll want to be sure to make other smart and health-inducing choices to your lifestyle. Getting enough sleep, getting some exercise, and engaging in ongoing self-reflection will only help solidify the habits for you.

Sleep Well and Stay Healthy—for Life

Scrimping on sleep may seem like a good way to squeeze in a few more productive hours into your busy day, but you may pay a hefty price with your health.

If you've noticed that you're hungrier and crave unhealthy foods when you don't get enough sleep, chalk it up to hormones. Studies show that when you sleep only four or five hours a night, the hunger hormone ghrelin spikes—so you feel really hungry the next day.

Plus, when you're sleep deprived, your body releases cortisol. When cortisol goes up, it tells your liver to release its stored glucose. But it also limits insulin. So, your blood sugar levels soar, making you crave foods, usually sugary carbs. Still other research has linked sleep deprivation to depression and anxiety, both prevalent in mid-life, as well as insulin resistance, which is a trigger for high blood pressure, heart disease, and type 2 diabetes.

One of the best ways to improve your sleep is to develop a sleep ritual—much like we did for our children when they were young. My daughters' bedtime routine included a taking bath and reading a story together before bedtime.

Do something similar for yourself now. A consistent nighttime ritual signals your brain and body to begin slowing down for the night. Some ideas for creating your own sleep ritual are as follows:

- Use white noise or earplugs, or silence your cell phone to reduce disruptions. Even better, place your cell phone in another room to avoid temptation.

- At night, reduce your exposure to bright and blue light (from electronics) 45 to 60 minutes before bedtime.
- Stick to a sleep schedule. Make a plan before your week gets busy. Look over your schedule and put together a sleep schedule that you can stick to. Go to bed and wake up at close to the same time each day. According to most medical guidelines, the optimal amount of sleep for most adults is seven to eight hours each night.
- Become a napper. Take a short nap when you can. If you work shifts and don't get enough sleep, napping can help you stay awake when you need to and avoid a sleep deficit. Even if you are a non-shift worker, don't deny yourself a 15- to 30-minute nap when you're weary. Any longer than that may interrupt your sleep schedule later that night.
- Avoid stimulants such as caffeine, alcohol, and nicotine at least six hours prior to bedtime. All three substances have the potential to impact the quality and length of your sleep.

Stay Active

If you started exercising or ramping up your workouts while embarking on the Galveston Diet, you'll want to maintain your exercise program, especially to manage your weight and other midlife symptoms.

Exercise is just so important now. It alters your body composition, increasing your lean muscle mass and shrinking your fat mass. Both changes help you maintain your new healthy weight.

It also improves your bone mineral density (BMD) and thus prevents or halts osteoporosis, the loss of bone mass that happens to be one of the biggest concerns as women enter menopause. In fact, the number one recommendation for preventing osteoporosis is regular exercise.

Those body aches and pains you've been dealing with? Exercise to the rescue. Most pain symptoms at this point in your life are associated with arthritis, hip pain, or lower back discomfort. It may seem counterintuitive, but when you work those "tough spots," the less they hurt in the long run.

I've talked in *The Galveston Diet* a lot about visceral fat and its dangers. As much as the three actions of the diet target this particularly hard-to-lose fat, regular exercise actually "moves" fat from your abdomen area and more evenly distributes it throughout your body.

Along with an anti-inflammatory diet, exercise protects against obesity-related diseases/complications, including type 2 diabetes, high blood pressure, certain types of cancer, fatty liver, and more. Regular physical activity also decreases your risk of developing breast cancer.

I love exercise, too, for how it makes me feel, mentally and emotionally. It boosts my mood and relieves stress. I feel more confident and more productive in my day-to-day life when I make and protect my commitment to move my body. It will help you, too.

The attitude to take is that it is never too late to become more active. If you're feeling overwhelmed by the prospect of adding exercise to your already busy lifestyle or if you're feeling defeated by prior years of inactivity, please don't give up. Any amount of exercise—a daily 20-minute walk, a half-hour yoga class, some strength training twice a week, a fun sport—that you can add to your life at any age will vastly improve your health and quality of life. The research is clear: few choices improve life and life expectancy more than exercise. So do it, and you'll feel terrific. Don't even consider it a choice!

Finally . . .

Remember that journal I asked you to keep at the start of this book? Well, take it out now and do some self-reflection. Note how far you've come. But look ahead, too. You have a lot of life yet to live. What do you want it to look like? How would you describe the life of your dreams?

Answer these questions with no limitations, as if you are guaranteed of not failing, but of having everything you want. Really allow yourself to express your desires, aspirations, and what you want to truly do with the rest of your life.

Your goals might be about fixing broken relationships . . . or making a difference in the world . . . or even more specific, like staying healthy and whole so you can enjoy your grandchildren someday (that's one of mine).

It's this kind of honesty and clarity that inspires us as to what's important on the journey ahead, and it helps us live with the hope that something wonderful is about to happen each and every day.

You're stepping into the most fulfilling season of your life. Enjoy it!

REFERENCES

Chapter 1

American Heart Association. 2015. "Menopause and Heart Disease." July 31. At www.heart.org.

Chopra, S., et al. 2019. "Weight Management Module for Perimenopausal Women: A Practical Guide for Gynecologists." *Journal of Mid-Life Health* 10: 165–72.

Dunneram, Y., et al. 2021. "Dietary Patterns and Age at Natural Menopause: Evidence from the UK Women's Cohort Study." *Maturitas* 143: 165–70.

Malabanan, A. O., and M. F. Holick. 2003. "Vitamin D and Bone Health in Postmenopausal Women." *Journal of Women's Health* 12: 151-56.

Saccomani, S., et al. 2017. "Does Obesity Increase the Risk of Hot Flashes among Midlife Women?: A Population-Based Study." *Menopause* 24: 1065–70.

Thurston, R. C., et al. 2008. "Abdominal Adiposity and Hot Flashes among Midlife Women." *Menopause* 15: 429–34.

Chapter 2

Aune, D., 2017. "Fruit and Vegetable Intake and the Risk of Cardiovascular Disease, Total Cancer and All-Cause Mortality: A Systematic Review and Dose-Response Meta-Analysis of Prospective Studies." *International Journal of Epidemiology* 46: 1029–56.

Ludwig, D., et al. 2020. "The Carbohydrate-Insulin Model: A Physiological Perspective on the Obesity Pandemic." *American Journal of Clinical Nutrition* 114: 1873–85.

Misra, S., and D. Mohanty. 2019. "Psychobiotics: A New Approach for Treating Mental Illness?" *Critical Reviews in Food Science and Nutrition* 59: 1230–36.

Pereira, M., et al. 2005. "Fast-Food Habits, Weight Gain, and Insulin Resistance (the CARDIA Study): 15-Year Prospective Analysis." *The Lancet* 365: 36–42.

Steptoe, A., et al. 2007. "The Effects of Tea on Psychophysiological Stress Responsivity and Post-Stress Recovery: A Randomised Double-Blind Trial." *Psychopharmacology* 190: 81–89.

Chapter 3

Egger, G. 1992. "The Case for Using Waist to Hip Ratio Measurements in Routine Medical Checks." *Medical Journal of Australia* 156: 280–85.

Chapter 4

Alirezaei, M., et al. 2010. "Short-Term Fasting Induces Profound Neuronal Autophagy." *Autophagy* 6: 702–10.

Baik, S. H., et al. 2020. "Intermittent Fasting Increases Adult Hippocampal Neurogenesis." *Brain and Behavior* 10: e01444.

Barnosky, A. R., et al. 2014. "Intermittent Fasting vs. Daily Calorie Restriction for Type 2 Diabetes Prevention: A Review of Human Findings." *Translational Research* 164: 302–11.

Collier, R. 2013. "Intermittent Fasting: The Science of Going Without." *Canadian Medical Association Journal* 185: e363–64.

de Cabo, R., and Mattson, M. P. 2019. "Effects of Intermittent Fasting on Health, Aging, and Disease." *New England Journal of Medicine* 381: 2541–51.

Guolin, L., et al. 2017. "Intermittent Fasting Promotes White Adipose Browning and Decreases Obesity by Shaping the Gut Microbiota." *Cell Metabolism* 26: 672–85.

Hartman, M. L., et al. 1992. "Augmented Growth Hormone (GH) Secretory Burst Frequency and Amplitude Mediate Enhanced GH Secretion during a Two-Day Fast in Normal Men." *Journal of Clinical Endocrinology and Metabolism* 74: 757–65.

Ho, K. Y., et al. 1988. "Fasting Enhances Growth Hormone Secretion and Amplifies the Complex Rhythms of Growth Hormone Secretion in Man." *Journal of Clinical Investigation* 81: 968–75.

Horne, B. D., et al. 2022. "Intermittent Fasting and Changes in Galectin-3: A Secondary Analysis of a Randomized Controlled Trial of Disease-Free Subjects." *Nutrition, Metabolism, and Cardiovascular Diseases* 32: 1538–48.

Jordan, S., et al. 2019. "Dietary Intake Regulates the Circulating Inflammatory Monocyte Pool." *Cell* 178: 1102–14.e17.

Klempel, M. C., et al. 2012. "Intermittent Fasting Combined with Calorie Restriction Is Effective for Weight Loss and Cardio-Protection in Obese Women." *Nutrition Journal* 11: 98.

Lean, M. Ej., et al. 2018. "Primary Care-Led Weight Management for Remission of Type 2 Diabetes (DiRECT): An Open-Label, Cluster-Randomised Trial." *The Lancet* 391: 541–51.

Longo, V. D., et al. 2015. "Interventions to Slow Aging in Humans: Are We Ready?" *Aging Cell* 14: 497–510.

Longo, V. D., and M. P. Mattson. 2014. "Fasting: Molecular Mechanisms and Clinical Applications." *Cell Metabolism* 19: 181–92.

Mattson, M., et al. 2014. "Meal Frequency and Timing in Health and Disease." *Proceedings of the National Academy of Sciences of the United States of America* 111: 16647–53.

Mattson, M. P., et al. 2017. "Impact of Intermittent Fasting on Health and Disease Processes." *Ageing Research Reviews* 39: 46–58.

Mindikoglu, A. L., et al. 2020. "Intermittent Fasting from Dawn to Sunset for 30 Consecutive Days Is Associated with Anticancer Proteomic Signature and Upregulates Key Regulatory Proteins of Glucose and Lipid Metabolism, Circadian Clock, DNA Repair, Cytoskeleton Remodeling, Immune System and Cognitive Function in Healthy Subjects." *Journal of Proteomics* 217: 103645.

Nair, P. M., and P. G. Khawale. 2016. "Role of Therapeutic Fasting in Women's Health: An Overview." *Journal of Mid-Life Health* 7: 61–4.

Natalucci, G., et al. 2005. "Spontaneous 24-h Ghrelin Secretion Pattern in Fasting Subjects: Maintenance of a Meal-Related Pattern." *European Journal of Endocrinology* 152: 845–50.

Patterson, R. E., et al. 2015. "Intermittent Fasting and Human Metabolic Health." *Journal of the Academy of Nutrition and Dietetics* 115: 1203–12.

Patterson, R. E., and D. D. Sears. 2017. "Metabolic Effects of Intermittent Fasting." *Annual Review of Nutrition* 37: 371–93.

Ravussin, E., et al. 2019. "Early Time-Restricted Feeding Reduces Appetite and Increases Fat Oxidation But Does Not Affect Energy Expenditure in Humans." *Obesity* 27: 1244–54.

Tinsley, G. M., and P. M. La Bounty. 2015. "Effects of Intermittent Fasting on Body Composition and Clinical Health Markers in Humans." *Nutrition Reviews* 73: 661–74.

Varady, K. A., et al. 2009. "Short-term Modified Alternate-day Fasting: A Novel Dietary Strategy for Weight Loss and Cardioprotection in Obese Adults." *American Journal of Clinical Nutrition* 90: 1138–43.

Wilkinson, M. J., et al. 2020. "Ten-Hour Time-Restricted Eating Reduces Weight, Blood Pressure, and Atherogenic Lipids in Patients with Metabolic Syndrome." *Cell Metabolism* 31: 92–104.e5.

Wegman, M. P., et al. 2015. "Practicality of Intermittent Fasting in Humans and Its Effect on Oxidative Stress and Genes Related to Aging and Metabolism." *Rejuvenation Research* 18: 162–72.

Chapter 5

Au, A., et al. 2016. "Estrogens, Inflammation and Cognition." *Frontiers in Neuroendocrinology* 40: 87–100.

Bosma-den Boer, M. M., et al. 2012. "Chronic Inflammatory Diseases Are Stimulated by Current Lifestyle: How Diet, Stress Levels and Medication Prevent Our Body from Recovering." *Nutrition & Metabolism* 9: 32.

Gambardella J., and G. Santulli. 2016. "Integrating Diet and Inflammation to Calculate Cardiovascular Risk." *Atherosclerosis* 253: 258–61.

Myles, I. A. 2014. "Fast Food Fever: Reviewing the Impacts of the Western Diet on Immunity." *Nutrition Journal* 13: 61.

Nettleton, J. A., et al. 2006. "Dietary Patterns Are Associated with Biochemical Markers of Inflammation and Endothelial Activation in the Multi-Ethnic Study of Atherosclerosis (MESA)." *American Journal of Clinical Nutrition* 83: 1369–79.

Rogero, M. M., and P. C. Calder. 2018. "Obesity, Inflammation, Toll-Like Receptor 4 and Fatty Acids." *Nutrients* 10: 432.

Sears, B., and C. Ricordi. 2011. "Anti-Inflammatory Nutrition as a Pharmacological Approach to Treat Obesity." *Journal of Obesity* 2011: 431985.

Serafini, M., and I. Peluso. 2016. "Functional Foods for Health: The Interrelated Antioxidant and Anti-Inflammatory Role of Fruits, Vegetables, Herbs, Spices and Cocoa in Humans." *Current Pharmaceutical Design* 22: 6701–15.

Shieh, A., et al. 2020. "Gut Permeability, Inflammation, and Bone Density Across the Menopause Transition." *JCI Insight* 5: e134092.

Zhu, F., et al. 2018. "Anti-inflammatory Effects of Phytochemicals from Fruits, Vegetables, and Food Legumes: A Review." *Critical Reviews in Food Science and Nutrition* 58: 1260–70.

Chapter 6

Arnold, K., et al. 2018. "Improving Diet Quality Is Associated with Decreased Inflammation: Findings from a Pilot Intervention in Postmenopausal Women with Obesity." *Journal of the Academy of Nutrition and Dietetics* 118: 2135–43.

Lennerz, B., and J. K. Lennerz. 2018. "Food Addiction, High-Glycemic-Index Carbohydrates, and Obesity." *Clinical Chemistry* 64: 64–71.

Lenoir, M., et al. 2007. "Intense Sweetness Surpasses Cocaine Reward." *PLoS ONE* 2: e698.

Madsen, H. B., and S. H. Ahmed. 2015. "Drug versus Sweet Reward: Greater Attraction to and Preference for Sweet versus Drug Cues." *Addiction Biology* 20: 433–44.

Seidelmann, S. B., et al. 2018. "Dietary Carbohydrate Intake and Mortality: A Prospective Cohort Study and Meta-Analysis." *Lancet Public Health* 3: e419–28.

Tabung, F. K., et al. 2015. "The Association between Dietary Inflammatory Index and Risk of Colorectal Cancer among Postmenopausal Women: Results from the Women's Health Initiative." *Cancer Causes Control* 26: 399–408.

Wise, P. M., et al. 2016. "Reduced Dietary Intake of Simple Sugars Alters Perceived Sweet Taste Intensity but Not Perceived Pleasantness." *American Journal of Clinical Nutrition* 103: 50–60.

Chapter 7

Abbasi, B., et al. 2012. "The Effect of Magnesium Supplementation on Primary Insomnia in Elderly: A Double-Blind Placebo-Controlled Clinical Trial." *Journal of Research in Medical Sciences* 17: 1161–69.

Bacciottini, L., et al. 2007. "Phytoestrogens: Food or Drug?" *Clinical Cases in Mineral and Bone Metabolism* 4: 123–30.

Barbagallo, M., et al. 2021. "Magnesium in Aging, Health and Diseases." *Nutrients* 13: 463.

Barnard, N. D., et al. 2021. "The Women's Study for the Alleviation of Vasomotor Symptoms (WAVS): A Randomized, Controlled Trial of a Plant-Based Diet and Whole Soybeans for Postmenopausal Women." *Menopause* 28: 1150–56.

Cangusso, L. M., et al. 2015. "Effect of Vitamin D Supplementation Alone on Muscle Function in Postmenopausal Women: A Randomized, Double-Blind, Placebo-Controlled Clinical Trial." *Osteoporosis International* 26: 2413–21.

Chacko, S. A., et al. 2010. "Relations of Dietary Magnesium Intake to Biomarkers of Inflammation and Endothelial Dysfunction in an Ethnically Diverse Cohort of Postmenopausal Women." *Diabetes Care* 33: 304–10.

Chen, S., et al. 2016. "Dietary Fibre Intake and Risk of Breast Cancer: A Systematic Review and Meta-Analysis of Epidemiological Studies." *Oncotarget* 7: 80980–89.

Cheng, Y. C., et al. 2020. "The Effect of Vitamin D Supplement on Negative Emotions: A Systematic Review and Meta-Analysis." *Depression and Anxiety* 37: 549–64.

Durosier-Izart, C., et al. 2017. "Peripheral Skeleton Bone Strength Is Positively Correlated with Total and Dairy Protein Intakes in Healthy Postmenopausal Women." *American Journal of Clinical Nutrition* 105: 513–25.

Durrant. L. R., et al. 2022. "Vitamins D_2 and D_3 Have Overlapping But Different Effects on the Human Immune System Revealed Through Analysis of the Blood Transcriptome." *Frontiers in Immunology* 13: 790444.

Estébanez, N., et al. 2018. "Vitamin D Exposure and Risk of Breast Cancer: A Meta-analysis." *Scientific Reports* 8: 9039.

Fowke, J. H., et al. 2000. "Brassica Vegetable Consumption Shifts Estrogen Metabolism in Healthy Postmenopausal Women." *Cancer Epidemiology, Biomarkers & Prevention* 9: 773–79.

Hairston, K. G., et al. 2012. "Lifestyle Factors and 5-Year Abdominal Fat Accumulation in a Minority Cohort: The IRAS Family Study." *Obesity* 20: 421–27.

Kim, J. M., and Y. J. Park. 2017. "Probiotics in the Prevention and Treatment of Postmenopausal Vaginal Infections: Review Article." *Journal of Menopausal Medicine* 23: 139–45.

Kroenke, C. H., et al. 2012. "Effects of a Dietary Intervention and Weight Change on Vasomotor Symptoms in the Women's Health Initiative." *Menopause* 19: 980–88.

Maalmi, H., et al. 2014. "Serum 25-hydroxyvitamin D Levels and Survival in Colorectal and Breast Cancer Patients: Systematic Review and Meta-Analysis of Prospective Cohort Studies." *European Journal of Cancer* 50: 1510–21.

Masoudi, A. N., et al. 2015. "Fatigue and Vitamin D Status in Iranian Female Nurses." *Global Journal of Health Science* 8: 196–202.

Mossavar-Rahmani, Y., et al. 2019. "Artificially Sweetened Beverages and Stroke, Coronary Heart Disease, and All-Cause Mortality in the Women's Health Initiative." *Stroke* 50: 555–62.

Orchard, T. S., et al. 2014. "Magnesium Intake, Bone Mineral Density, and Fractures: Results from the Women's Health Initiative Observational Study." *American Journal of Clinical Nutrition* 99: 926–33.

Parra, D. et al. 2008. "A Diet Rich in Long Chain Omega-3 Fatty Acids Modulates Satiety in Overweight and Obese Volunteers during Weight Loss." *Appetite* 51: 676–80.

Parazzini, F. 2015. "Resveratrol, Tryptophanum, Glycine and Vitamin E: A Nutraceutical Approach to Sleep Disturbance and Irritability in Peri- and Post-Menopause." *Minerva Ginecologica* 67: 1–5.

Piuri, G., et al. 2021. "Magnesium in Obesity, Metabolic Syndrome, and Type 2 Diabetes." *Nutrients* 13: 320.

Rondanelli, M., et al. 2021. "An Update on Magnesium and Bone Health." *Biometals* 34: 715–36.

Santoro, N., et al. 2015. "Menopausal Symptoms and Their Management." *Endocrinology and Metabolism Clinics of North America* 44: 497–515.

Zhang, Y. Y., et al. 2017. "Efficacy of Omega-3 Polyunsaturated Fatty Acids Supplementation in Managing Overweight and Obesity: A Meta-Analysis of Randomized Clinical Trials." *Journal of Nutrition, Health, and Aging* 21: 187–92.

Chapter 10

Ayas, N. T., et al. 2003. "A Prospective Study of Sleep Duration and Coronary Heart Disease in Women." *Archives of Internal Medicine* 163: 205–209.

Bayon, V., et al. 2014. "Sleep Debt and Obesity." *Annals of Medicine* 46: 264–72.

Hanson, J. A., and M. R. Huecker. "Sleep Deprivation." In StatPearls. Treasure Island, FL: StatPearls Publishing, 2022.

Steger, F. L, et al. 2021. "Intermittent and Continuous Energy Restriction Result in Similar Weight Loss, Weight Loss Maintenance, and Body Composition Changes in a 6 Month Randomized Pilot Study." *Clinical Obesity* 11: e12430.

RESOURCES

The following resources are those I recommend to help your journey on The Galveston Diet be even more successful.

Books

This Is Your Brain on Food by Dr. Uma Naiboo

The Intermittent Fasting Revolution: The Science of Optimizing Health and Enhancing Performance by Mark P. Mattson

Hooked by Michael Moss

Mini Habits for Weight Loss by Stephen Guise

Untamed by Glennon Doyle

The Obesity Code: Unlocking the Secrets of Weight Loss by Dr. Jason Fung

The Diabetes Code: Prevent and Reverse Type 2 Diabetes Naturally by Dr. Jason Fung

In Defense of Food: An Eater's Manifesto by Michael Pollan

The Longevity Solution: Rediscovering Centuries-Old Secrets to a Healthy, Long Life by Dr. James DiNicolantonio and Dr. Jason Fung

Atomic Habits: An Easy & Proven Way to Build Good Habits & Break Bad Ones by James Clear
Salt Sugar Fat: How the Food Giants Hooked Us by Michael Moss
Metabolical: The Lure and the Lies of Processed Food, Nutrition, and Modern Medicine by Robert Lustig, MD, MSL
Soundtracks: The Surprising Solution to Overthinking by Jon Acuff
Lifespan: Why We Age—and Why We Don't Have To by Dr. David Sinclair and Matthew LaPlante

Podcasts

Weight Loss for Food-Lovers
You Are Not Broken by Kelly Casperson, MD
The Life Coach School
Unlocking Us with Brené Brown
We Can Do Hard Things with Glennon Doyle
The Improvement Project
Tara Brach

Websites and Social Media

Doctor Referral Program: www.galvestondiet.com/recommended-physicians/
Galveston for Life Community: www.community.galvestondiet.com/home
The Galveston Diet Perimenopause Quiz: www.galvestondiet.com/perimenopause-quiz/
The Galveston Diet Nutritional Anti-Inflammation Quiz: www.galvestondiet.com/nutritional-anti-inflammation-quiz/
The Galveston Diet Supplements: www.shop.galvestondiet.com/
The Galveston Diet Website: www.galvestondiet.com
The Galveston Diet Blogs: www.galvestondiet.com/blogs
The Galveston Diet Supplements: shop.galvestondiet.com
The Galveston Diet Workout: www.galvestondiet.com

Facebook: The Galveston Diet Mary Claire Haver, MD
Instagram: thegalvestondiet
YouTube: @Mary Claire Haver, MD
TikTok: @drmaryclaire
Cronometer for The Galveston Diet: www.cronometer.com/galveston/

ACKNOWLEDGMENTS

I have many people to thank for helping me write this book and, with it, for opening the door to an even wider audience. I am grateful to:

My patients who inspire me every day.

My followers who taught me to be a better advocate and inspired me to fill in the gaps of my training and knowledge.

My family: Chris Haver, for his unflagging belief in me; Katherine Haver, for keeping me honest with her nutrition science degree; and Madeline Haver, who keeps me honest on social media and all aspects of motherhood.

The early volunteers who tested the program and provided so much feedback.

The early contributors to the program: Cara Coza, Heidi Seigel, Stephanie Vasut, Stephanie Haver, Leah Pastor, and Dr. Alison Warlick.

Those who inspired me: Dr. Kelly Casperson, Dr. Shannon Clark, Dr. David Sinclair and Dr. Tony Youn.

The Galveston Diet Team: Jen Pearson, Margaret Walsh, Michelle

Jones, Ashley Simon, Victoria Thomas, Dawn Drogosch, Jamie Hadley, Sara Joseph, Zach Toth, Ani Hadjinian, Kathy Champagne, Cody Wright, and Judy Corsmeier.

My publishing team: Marnie Cochran, Heather Jackson, and Maggie Greenwood-Robinson.

INDEX

ABOUT THE AUTHOR

Mary Claire Haver, MD, is a board-certified OB-GYN and a Certified Culinary Medicine Specialist in medical nutrition. With a thriving practice in Houston, Texas, she has delivered thousands of babies, completed thousands of well-woman exams, and regularly counsels patients through their health issues. She developed her groundbreaking weight-loss protocol as an online subscriber program, through which she has helped more than 100,000 women lose weight, burn fat, and get in shape permanently. Dr. Haver lives with her husband and two daughters in Galveston, Texas.

www.galvestondiet.com

@thegalvestondiet